Susan Sontag as Metaphor

A Docuplay by the Author of

The Chronic Fatigue Syndrome

Epidemic Cover-up

Charles Ortleb

HHV-6 University Press, Salem, Massachusetts

PRINTED IN THE UNITED STATES OF AMERICA

ISBN: 9781652012023

10 9 8 7 6 5 4 3 2 1
First Edition

"The writer's first job is not to have opinions but to tell the truth . . . and refuse to be an accomplice of lies and misinformation."

-- Susan Sontag

Author's Note

This play begins with an interview I did with Susan Sontag that was conducted in late 1973 and published in a magazine called *Out* in 1974. All the dialogue from the interview in the play is drawn from that interview. Some of the monologue in the second half of the play is based on *The Chronic Fatigue Syndrome Epidemic Cover-up*.

CHARACTERS

YOUNG ORTLEB: Twenty-three, with thick blond hair, dressed in 70s casual clothing.

OLD ORTLEB: Seventy, without thick blond hair, dressed in white shirt and tie.

SUSAN SONTAG: Forty, dressed in a black turtleneck and black slacks.

The stage is divided into two sections. The opening interview takes place in a loft which is Stage Left. The loft is white and minimalist with a maximum number of books on a bookcase that runs across the entire wall. SUSAN SONTAG sits in a black La-Z-Boy and YOUNG ORTLEB sits on the floor facing her. On the table beside him is a small tape recorder. SUSAN SONTAG is smoking. Someplace above them "1973" is projected. On Stage Right there is a large editor-in-chief kind of desk at which OLD ORTLEB sits. There is a screen behind him that will project images from the publications, Christopher Street *and* New York Native. *Above the desk "2020" is projected. Above the players, at the back of the stage, there is a projection of the all the titles of Sontag's works. The most prominent one is* AIDS and Its Metaphors.

Throughout the interview, YOUNG ORTLEB and SUSAN SONTAG stare at each other. They do not react to OLD ORTLEB who makes comments about them from decades in the future. He looks over at them every time he makes a comment about their interview.

Before the curtain goes up, OLD ORTLEB walks out to center stage with a white rose in his hand and speaks directly to the audience.

OLD ORTLEB: (*To the audience.*) On Sunday, December 5, 2005, when I read David Rieff's description of the death of his mother, Susan Sontag, in the *New York Times Magazine*, I was gobsmacked. I couldn't believe that one of the world's most famous and most photogenic public intellectuals, had a wretched and troubling death. I think I speak for you, too, when I say it was not the death any of us would have imagined her having. There was something darkly disturbing and downright cockamamie about her death. Even in the last days, when her body was wracked with cancer and the horrifying side effects of the draconian medical interventions she had asked for, she seemed genuinely surprised that she was going to die. Maybe we are all mistaken in our notion that intellectuals have thought death through deeply and stoically accept its inevitability. She seemed to think that she was some kind of supernatural exception; that her death, the death of the great Susan Sontag, was unthinkable, unacceptable, some big mistake. While there are those who might see her very fraught death as an expression of a valiant will to live, I'm afraid that I view it as the harrowing death of a sociopathic soul, a very fucked-up woman. How dare I say that? I knew Susan Sontag personally. Or, I thought I did.

The curtain opens and he walks to the desk with the images of covers of New York Native *behind it. He sits down.*

OLD ORTLEB: *(To the audience.)* The last time I saw her, Susan Sontag hugged me and said, "You're very real to me." It seemed like an affirmative thing to say, but it also struck me as very odd and puzzled me for decades. In my seventy years, she is the only person who has ever said those precise words to me. That was in 1987. But our story begins fourteen years before when I interviewed Susan Sontag in 1973 for a new magazine called *Out*. "The Gay Perspective" was the subtitle of the magazine. It may not have been the only gay magazine an interview with Sontag ever appeared in, but it was the first. And the only one to put her on the cover, I think. The issue that came out in April of 1974 was the second and, unfortunately, final issue of *Out*, a magazine we had high hopes for. It was started by a handful of former members of the Gay Activist Alliance in New York. We wanted to be a gay version of *Ms. Magazine*, but the small amount of money raised for it didn't go very far. The starstruck introduction is like finding my embarrassing gullible youth returning to shore in a bottle. (*Holds a copy of Out and begins reading from it.*) In the introduction I wrote, "I first encountered Susan Sontag on paperback bookrack in Lawrence, Kansas. It was the face on the cover of *Against Interpretation* that did it. The eyes looking over to the left signaled a different perspective. The mouth was sensuous and serious at the same time. Inside, I found enough dazzling authority to let the bibliographies of Sartre and De Beauvoir pause and let someone else influence me for a while. It was the summer before the summer I came out, a time when arguments start to brew in one's head, broad generalizations about being open to experience, i.e. gay. Here was this delightfully arrogant, hip woman at the top of the mountain (New York) ruling on the most important creations on earth (books and movies) who recognized and defended the contributions of gay people to the arts. The summer of self-justification was also the summer of over-generalization. Therefore, it seemed to me that being gay was the source of *all* major creativity, and anyone who didn't recognize that, anyone who couldn't get into Jack Smith's *Flaming Creatures*, Norman O. Brown's theories, and Camp itself, was, well probably from Lawrence, Kansas. I was one of those people who thought that reading Sontag, *The New York Times Book Review*, and the *Village Voice* makes you a New Yorker before you set one foot in New York. Other Sontag works, more illusions about New York, and more authentic reasons for being gay passed through my head between that summer and November when word spread around the Gay Academic Union conference that 'Susan Sontag is here.' Drop everything. Chance of a lifetime. I just walk right up to her. She looks great, like the Mrs. Robinson of the Seventies. I tell her I've written her two letters that I have never mailed. She tells me I should have mailed them. I ask her for an interview. She says yes. A week later I am in the most ascetic penthouse on the Upper West Side. One of the walls is covered with books. On another wall is a Maoist poster. I'm not sure whether it's camp or serious or both. She sits back on the one piece of furniture in her living room, a black La-Z-Boy. I sit on the floor beside her thinking that now I am officially in New York."

YOUNG ORTLEB: (*Looking at the tape recorder.*). Okay, I think this thing is going to work now. (*Pause.*) In your piece on Paul Goodman, written soon after his death, you mentioned that you were trying to live a year without books. What precipitated that?

OLD ORTLEB: (*Looking over at them.*) Isn't he cute? I bet she thinks he is hot. He's in a total fanboy trance.

SUSAN SONTAG: My first novel was published in 1963. That means that it's ten years now, that I have been visible as a writer and have had to deal with people's reactions to what I write. I'm objective about my work, I think. I don't disavow it, but I hope to become a better, somewhat different, kind of writer. And changing as a writer, of course means growing as a person. It involves changing where I live, the way I live.

OLD ORTLEB: I wanted her life. I wanted her apartment. I wanted her books. I wanted her hair. Little can they imagine in this shiny New York City moment of acolyte-meets-icon that the story of the century is on the horizon and will soon engulf both of them.

SUSAN SONTAG: Doing without books for a while is a symbolic renunciation—I feel like Samurai who has cut off his top knot—that's helpful for me. I need to make myself uncomfortable. I'm not a person who is ever comfortable. I'm too puritanical, I suppose. Still, as one gets older, older in any sense (one is always older than one was before), there is a tendency to be more comfortable and settle into the options that one already has or has managed to create. Anyway, I'm just at the beginning of the work that will come out of the disruption of my habits, a second decade of work.

YOUNG ORTLEB: Do you have any intuition of what the character of that work is going to be?

SUSAN SONTAG: Wiser and more direct.

OLD ORTLEB. *(To the audience.)* With at least one big exception.

YOUNG ORTLEB: In 1965 you spoke of "the new sensibility" which is "pluralistic, high speed, and hectic"; and in 1973 in "Debriefing," in *American Review,* we find lines like: "We know more than we can use. Look at all the stuff I've got in my head: rockets and Venetian churches, David Bowie and Diderot, Nuoc Nam and Big Mac's, sunglasses and orgasms." Has the new sensibility had enough?

SUSAN SONTAG: First of all, I wrote about the new sensibility in an essay and "Debriefing" was fiction. But "Debriefing" is very important for me because it is an autobiographical story. It's only the second piece of fiction I've ever written that is also autobiographical; the very first is a story published in *The Atlantic Monthly* in April 1973, called "Project for a Trip to China." The two stories are recent work. But I reached a turning point in 1968 when I came back from Hanoi and started the book about my trip. That was the first thing that I ever wrote in which I felt that I was describing myself. The other voices in the fiction I'd written up to then were masks. I don't have anything against masks.

OLD ORTLEB: You can say that again.

SUSAN SONTAG: As Oscar Wilde says, masks are often more interesting and more true than faces. Nevertheless, I had been hiding as well as making myself braver with my masks. You know, the camp essay is dedicated to Oscar Wilde.

OLD ORTLEB: He might be rolling over in his gay grave.

SUSAN SONTAG: When I wrote it in 1964, I had just read the big edition of his *Letters* and was tremendously moved by his intelligence and his moral sense. Wilde is underrated as a serious presence in our culture. People are misled by elegant smart-ass tone; they don't see his originality, much less the fact that some of his ideas parallel Nietzsche's. Now, I suppose, he's remembered mostly as a gay martyr.

OLD ORTLEB: Not something you ever had to worry about.

YOUNG ORTLEB: What, exactly, happened when you were writing *Trip to Hanoi*?

SUSAN SONTAG: Until 1968, pretty much from the time I started publishing, my choices as a writer were guided mostly by a notion of the inherent value of what was "interesting." (That's one of the notions I'm questioning now.) Wearing masks as a writer served "the interesting." Masks give one entry to many different places, to the complexity of experience. And I found that many things that stimulated me were not well known, at least seldom discussed in print.

OLD ORTLEB: Like, uh . . . lesbianism?

SUSAN SONTAG: So, after *The Benefactor*, I started writing essays about those things. Then an inevitable evolution took place in relation to my own work, particularly concerning the first person—who was talking when I wrote "I." Politics seemed to require that I speak with an "I" that wasn't masked; for it was anything but "the interesting" which was at stake in the American aggression in Vietnam. I had to say "I" and mean, simply, "I" precisely because the book (actually, it was a very long essay) wasn't about me; it was about the Vietnamese. But having made the move for political—or moral—reasons, I got into a crisis about the rest of my writing. It was hard to go back to the complicated self-protective "I," the "I" that wasn't really me but projected itself into various experiences and tastes that I didn't think I had to take full responsibility for. And I virtually stopped writing for a couple of years, except for the scripts of the two movies I directed in Sweden in 1968 and 1970.

OLD ORTLEB: And film history, thus, was made.

SUSAN SONTAG: Filmmaking was a way of not having to say "I" at all, not having to deal with that question because *I* wasn't in the movie. (I mean, that's how I thought about it then.) At the end of 1970, I left Stockholm and went to Paris, where I went through a miserable year in which I didn't know whether to make another film or go back to writing. So, I didn't do either. And the new writing had been very different. The "I" is much more me. It's not the sort of confessional writing that has become so fashionable lately. Everybody wants to come out one way or another, whatever their closet may be. I do, too, in my own way. I want to have a more direct contact with my own "I."

OLD ORTLEB: Breaking news! Susan Sontag's "I" almost came out in the gay magazine *Out* in 1974. Close, but no cigar.

YOUNG ORTLEB: And the "I" of "Debriefing"?

SUSAN SONTAG: Yes, it's much closer to "me." It is me in the sense that I feel most things that the "I" in the story says, as well as many things which aren't in the story. To get back to your original question. In the "I" of that story—you're absolutely right—I was expressing discontent, a sense of confinement with the avidity which had flourished in the 1960s. You're right in seeing that theme in "Debriefing" as a comment on "One Culture and the New Sensibility." But because one is the argument of an essay and the other is in the context of a story, the clash isn't direct. I don't feel that I've really said what I think now until the response is in essay form. In a year or so, I hope to write an essay about the problem of sensibility in modern culture as such (that's what I was really trying to get at in the essay on camp) and about culture overload, in what way it's liberating and in what way it's destructive.

OLD ORTLEB: She never wrote an essay on closet lesbian sensibility in modern culture. Now that would have been a doozy. But wait a minute. Maybe all her work is the expression of the closet lesbian sensibility.

SUSAN SONTAG: I've started saying a little of it in the essays I've been doing on photography for *The New York Review of Books*, both the first one and the second one, which is mainly about Diane Arbus. I had met Diane Arbus—I don't mention that in the essay—in 1964 or '65, and saw some of her photographs. (This was before she had her first show.) And I loved her work. There was none of the reserve that I felt last year when I saw the retrospective at the Museum of Modern Art. If I had written about Diane Arbus in the mid-60s, it would have been a completely enthusiastic appraisal. And the fact that the essay I ended up writing criticizes some of the attitudes that lie behind her work, and the current enthusiasm for her work, illustrates my evolution. But it's terribly complicated. The fact that I didn't finish the essay until a year after I saw the MOMA show testifies to the conflict I feel about these matters. The Arbus essay was hard to write. And I don't want to take positions unless I'm really sure I believe what I am saying. I think now, looking back, that I didn't really believe all the things I said in the essays I wrote in the 1960s.

OLD ORTLEB: Only in the 1960s?

SUSAN SONTAG: So, writing now, instead of getting easier is getting harder and harder. I sweat over every sentence.

OLD ORTLEB: Maybe not enough.

YOUNG ORTLEB: To read through your early essays was like going up, and to read 'Debriefing" and the Arbus piece is to come down. The mood has utterly changed.

OLD ORTLEB: You ain't seen nothin' yet.

SUSAN SONTAG: Oh, I'm not going down. I know what you're saying though. There was a kind of euphoria that I felt in the mid-60s that came from political naivete and a somewhat adolescent embrace of the pleasures of cultural consumerism.

OLD ORTLEB: Party Pooper!

SUSAN SONTAG: I don't see how anyone can feel euphoric now in that way, anyone who's aware of what's going on. The mid 60s was actually a very simple moment—a time of opening to all kinds of experience. And that was good. Now we have to move to a more complex sense of things and integrate our discoveries with a less self-centered view of history.

OLD ORTLEB Uh-oh.

SUSAN SONTAG: Personally, I'm still euphoric. Because I'm alive and I'm grateful to be alive.

OLD ORTLEB: You go girl! You don't have a clue that you will have cancer in two years.

YOUNG ORTLEB: I'd like to talk to about your essay on camp. Because, fortunately or unfortunately, most people identify you with that.

SUSAN SONTAG: Unfortunately for me.

YOUNG ORTLEB: Why?

SUSAN SONTAG. That essay has really been an albatross. But when I look back at my work it remains one of the things that I like best. I still think it's good. It was rather easy to write, but then writing used to be altogether easier, less problematic for me than it is now. As I sat down to write "Notes on Camp," I wondered why Auden hadn't written it. It seemed to me a subject just begging to be written about by several people who might have done it as well or better than I, that it was by some kind of odd oversight that this essay had not yet been written. I never thought that I was saying anything particularly new.

OLD ORTLEB: Good to know.

SUSAN SONTAG: What did seem to me to be original was the form and tone of the essay. You can imagine my astonishment when people took it as my discovery. Some people actually thought I had invented the word. And practically everyone assumed that I was describing my own sensibility, that I was championing camp—when, God help me, it was one just one, of my masks.

OLD ORTLEB: God forbid anyone thought you were describing *your own* sensibility.

SUSAN SONTAG: I was dismayed when it became so well known, to the detriment of other things I had written. And—I was pretty naïve then—I was surprised and embarrassed by the commercial exploitation of the essay. Remember, it was published in 1964 in *Partisan Review*; and, when I was writing it, I thought of it as destined for that audience and that audience only, the fans of Lionel Trilling and Hannah Arendt and Harold Rosenberg.

OLD ORTLEB: Not every latent homosexual in America?

SUSAN SONTAG: I never imagined that something in *Partisan Review* would immediately get picked up and made into an industry. Right away, there were lots of articles written about it—in *Time*, *Life*, and so on. Publishers wrote me with ideas for books on camp. One of the big networks proposed a television special or a series. I was appalled.

OLD ORTLEB. Closet alert.

SUSAN SONTAG: I didn't want to be identified with camp. I only wanted to be identified with my own essay. I'd said all I could think of to say about camp in that essay.

YOUNG ORTLEB: But you think the essay stands up.

SUSAN SONTAG: Yes, I think it names a real thing. The point of "Notes on Camp" was to analyze a type of sensibility which, though mainly identified with homosexuals (the word itself is homosexual slang), is fairly widespread. It is not the major sensibility, the classical sensibility.

OLD ORTLEB: The classical white male heterosexual sensibility?

SUSAN SONTAG: It's a kind of alternative sensibility. But it's a valid one, and not limited to people with a particular sexual taste. I was trying to take camp out of the closet in another sense of "out of the closet," not to keep it as a gay-identified sensibility.

OLD ORTLEB. So many closets, so little time.

SUSAN SONTAG: Camp is a lot more than just something that operates as the self-justification of an oppressed, defensive sexual minority. Though that's *one* of the uses of camp. That's the context in which I compare homosexuals and Jews—a comparison Proust made, with a different point in mind, fifty years ago.

OLD ORTLEB. Proust and Sontag invented intersectionality.

YOUNG ORTLEB: In the Goodman piece you mention that there is a terrible mean resentment toward someone who tries to do a lot of things. You've tried to do a lot of things. Have you experienced a lot of resentment?

SUSAN SONTAG: I don't want to complain. Because I have also received a lot of encouragement.

OLD ORTLEB: Lucky you.

SUSAN SONTAG: Still the climate in this country *isn't* very helpful to people who want to spread themselves around.

OLD ORTLEB: Tell me about it, girlfriend.

SUSAN SONTAG: Goodman did suffer from that for many years until his work came together in one convenient way, when he published *Growing Up Absurd* in 1960. Because I belong to a completely different generation, I never had the problem that he had—working for years and years with a very, very tiny audience.

OLD ORTLEB: Try publishing a gay literary magazine. Then you'll really see what a tiny audience is.

SUSAN SONTAG: I started publishing in the '60s, a time when there was (as I found out) a rapid media amplification of whatever people were doing. People who would formerly have been just "little magazine writers"—and would have stayed that way for most, if not all, of their careers—suddenly became big names. But after the first years, when people were generous, I got hit hard in some reviews and articles on me.

OLD ORTLEB: Pray tell.

SUSAN SONTAG: It started with the publication of my second novel, *Death Kit.* In 1967 I realized that things were changing and that whatever I wrote from then on would be damned or dismissed by a fair number of people, mainly because by that time there was a certain crystallization of resentment against the range of my activities and the place that I had unselfconsciously put myself. Much of the resistance I've encountered in the last five or six years seems derived from an image that's been established about me, rather than from a reaction to the work itself. That's a common problem for a writer, of course. Either you encounter it in the beginning, or you encounter it later on. People put you in a box. I landed in a number of boxes which I didn't like.

OLD ORTLEB: Did someone say, "lesbian box?"

SUSAN SONTAG: One was "intellectual"—almost always a put-down in America, especially for a woman. Another was "chic" or "avant-garde." It's a problem but it doesn't help much to think about it.

When you first start to write you're not dealing with other people's preconceptions, misconceptions, and expectations. Then the feedback starts. And eventually the image that people have of you becomes, or can become, one of your motives for writing this rather than that—because you want to clear up what you think is a misconception. That's very dangerous, because you may have a misconception about other people's misconceptions. You may not even be reading correctly the response that you get. The relation to the public, to one's constituency as a writer, is very mysterious. You can't ignore it because that would be arrogant and stupid; but you can't pay too much attention to it either. For one thing, the information you have is very partial. Reviews are mostly what I have to go on. But who's writing the reviews?

YOUNG ORTLEB: Don't you meet many of your readers?

SUSAN SONTAG: Some, sure. And most people I meet say, within the first fifteen minutes, and as a compliment, "You're much nicer than I imagined." I guess I really got carried away with those masks!

YOUNG ORTLEB: Oh, you were exactly what I imagined.

OLD ORTLEB: *Then*, anyway.

SUSAN SONTAG: But you're a good reader; I can tell that from your questions. You're very tuned in to what I'm doing.

OLD ORTLEB. This lovefest is getting out of hand.

YOUNG ORTLEB: How about the way the reviewers handled you as a filmmaker?

OLD ORTLEB: Looks like the honeymoon is over.

SUSAN SONTAG: I think some people did feel, when I started making films, "Who does she think she is?" I'm not saying the films aren't flawed; they are. But certain reviews were terribly hostile—for example, the review of *Brother Carl* in the *Village Voice*. The whole review was a very personal attack on me. (I'd never even heard of, much less met, the reviewer.) The film was dismissed in one line. Listen, I don't want to complain about reviews. Personal attacks hurt, but I have to stand my ground—like anyone else who does things in public—and try to be brave.

YOUNG ORTLEB: The idea of a miracle is very important in *Brother Carl*. Why are you using a religious term in a secular context?

SUSAN SONTAG: Well, I believe in miracles. The problem is that all words were originally religious words. What I mean by "miracle" is that things do happen which are in some ways unmerited or unearned, which defy all odds. This has been used as evidence of the supernatural, but I'm not using it as evidence of anything, except that more is possible than most people imagine and that it makes sense to dare to orient your life around the unlikely. The only interesting events, finally, are miracles—those moments when things leap out of themselves. That's what most of great literature is about. But most books that feel modern have been about a miracle not happening. *Madame Bovary*, for instance. It's about somebody wanting something different but being absolutely incapable of producing it because of the corruption and insignificance, finally, of the heroine's circumstances and imagination. All that's told with the greatest sympathy, but, nevertheless, Madame Bovary's imagination is corrupt. Her folly is inspired by vulgar models which can never support her fantasies and make them come true. So, she's a dupe, and she doesn't understand what's she's doing.

OLD ORTLEB: (*To the audience.*) Like when somebody wrote *AIDS and Its Metaphors*?

SUSAN SONTAG: A lot of art in the last hundred years has been about people not managing to do what they want to because they haven't made the proper kind of spiritual efforts. That's what attracts me in works of art and in life—the absence or presence of a miracle. I don't think of it as something religious. Though you could explain it in religious terms, any terms which go beyond a demeaning and reductive analysis of human existence have to take account of the unpredictable and wholly extraordinary. But I don't mean to suggest that all miracles are good. Hitler was also a kind of miracle.

OLD ORTLEB: Here we go.

SUSAN SONTAG: The phenomenon of Hitler is not just the result of the defeat of Germany in the First World War, the weakness of the Weimar Republic, the economic chaos of the 1920s, and so on. Somebody like Hitler isn't just the sum total of his circumstances. He was an evil genius. And I don't believe that Nazism would have existed without Hitler—some form of fascism, most likely, but not Nazism.

YOUNG ORTLEB: In your recent questionnaire in *Partisan Review*, you talk about how language expresses the sexist order. And in the article on Camus, in *Against Interpretation*, we find you saying that all great writers are either husbands or lovers. Does that hold for women?

SUSAN SONTAG: Don't remind me! I would never say that now. It's certainly rather ridiculous for a writer who is a woman to participate, even if inadvertently, in promoting the assumption that all writers are men. I've always tried to be careful about these things, but there I just fell into the trap. You know, that essay—I think I wrote it in 1964—isn't really about Camus. It's about responses to writers. That some writers are admired because they are so responsible and central, which other writers are admired because they're so far out and take so many unreasonable risks. Camus versus Rimbaud, for instance. But I regret the image.

YOUNG ORTLEB: In that questionnaire in *Partisan Review*, you say that "women who make a common front with men to bring about their mutual liberation" are pulling "a veil across the harsh realities of the power relations that determine all dialogue between the sexes." Does this hold for all men—or are any distinctions to be made about gay men?

OLD ORTLEB: Somebody call 911.

SUSAN SONTAG: Of course, there are men, some of them gay, who understand and are sympathetic to feminism. The point I was trying to make was a practical one, about what women need to do to raise their own level of consciousness. Women have to learn to do everything themselves, because the sexual division of labor has unfitted women—more precisely, trained women to think and act as if they were unfit—to perform many adult roles. So, there is a danger, if women and even the best-intentioned men work together prematurely, that they'll maintain some of the traditional sex role distinctions. It's hard for women to unlearn the habits of deferring to men, trying to please men, passing on the physically demanding or dangerous tasks to men. Women have to gain self-confidence, but that only comes through concrete experience of running things themselves and taking responsibility for their mistakes. That's why I'm in favor of all-women groups. By the way, I'm not as optimistic as you seem to be about gay men.

OLD ORTLEB: Fasten your seatbelts. It's going to be a bumpy night.

SUSAN SONTAG: Many of them could hardly be more sexist. In fact, their being gay is partly an expression of hatred for women.

OLD ORLEB: Say what? Here we go.

SUSAN SONTAG: But younger gay men, at least many who identify with the Gay Movement, certainly seem less misogynistic than the older ones.

OLD ORTLEB: There is nothing more misogynistic than an old Miss Thing.

YOUNG ORTLEB: So, you don't see much in common between Gay Liberation and Women's Liberation?

SUSAN SONTAG: I do, in the sense that potentially gay men should be able to understand the feminist argument very well.

OLD ORTLEB: I don't know if gay men even understand the gay argument very well.

SUSAN SONTAG: But gay men have to work out in their own heads why they're gay.

OLD ORTLEB: Sounds like a plan. That's certainly the pot calling the kettle gay.

SUSAN SONTAG: Every erotic choice is also a political choice, a comment about conventional sex roles. Often a protest. Everybody has the capacity for homosexual feelings and homosexual relations.

OLD ORTLEB: Everybody, Susan?

SUSAN SONTAG: But only some people choose to live out these feelings, whereas the majority don't at all. That some people actually do choose this sexual option, despite all the sexual penalties, often has more to do with their feelings about sex roles than with a direct sexual need.

OLD ORTLEB: Yes, the gay male community is a hotbed of political theorizing about sex roles. In gay bars, the sound of it is deafening.

SUSAN SONTAG: Certainly, this is true of almost all gay women I know, and of many gay men. I think most gay women are gay, mainly, because they couldn't stand to be shut up in the traditional women's roles and women's options. The deep basis for their sexual choice was a moral protest against the standards of second-class adulthood implied by the behavior of heterosexual women in relationship to men.

OLD ORTLEB: Sexual choice as moral protest? No wonder, back in the day, so many lesbians were ex-nuns.

SUSAN SONTAG: I don't mean they actually were, in all cases, freer. But the choice came out of a yearning for more autonomy than our society grants women. That's why I think—or hope—that homosexuality is evolving. If roles become less polarized and it's acceptable for men to have qualities and feelings and kinds of behavior which were hitherto stereotyped, and put down as "feminine"—and the other way around—one of the main reasons for, and advantages of, being homosexual would vanish.

OLD ORTLEB: Presto-change-o! No more camp! No more Cherry Grove!

SUSAN SONTAG: Homosexuality would become more purely an erotic choice. I think this evolution would promote bisexuality and weaken the need to be exclusively homosexual.

OLD ORTLEB: 47 years later, I'm still waiting for that tsunami of bisexuality. I mean the real kind, not the Upper West Side theoretical kind.

YOUNG ORTLEB: But still, isn't the biggest problem the people who remain exclusively heterosexuals?

OLD ORTLEB: Yeah, the holdouts!

SUSAN SONTAG: They're the problem because they're the majority. But if it involves repression for people to be exclusively heterosexual, the same is true for the sexual minority. Gay people have to repress their heterosexuality, though their reasons are very different from the reasons the straight majority repress their homosexual feelings.

OLD ORTLEB. Manhattan must be the capital of repressed heterosexuality. It's an epidemic on Broadway. Show me a showtune and I'll show you a repressed heterosexual.

SUSAN SONTAG: I have a good friend in his mid-forties who has been gay all his life, except for affair with a girl in college. He's always been attracted to women as well as men. But he feels threatened, not in a sexual way—he's confident he could function sexually—but by the specter of conformity, his idea of the psychological and social demands women would make on him. He sees himself becoming like his father, or some boring, unimaginative heterosexual male in his family. So, he's always repressed his desire for women, because he is convinced that to be gay is to be freer.

OLD ORTLEB: That's refreshing. It's dad's fault.

YOUNG ORTLEB: How strongly are your ideas on androgyny based on Norman O. Brown's ideas?

OLD ORTLEB: Show-off!

SUSAN SONTAG: They're not. I don't feel influenced by him at all. Brown's idea of androgyny remains on a very abstract level. I don't feel the cutting edge of real social criticism. For me, androgyny has a function—to get people out of their traps. Men can cry. Women can defend themselves physically. It's not some kind of mythic sexual idea for me, but a concrete form of liberation.

YOUNG ORTLEB. What about Jack Smith's film, *Flaming Creatures*?

SUSAN SONTAG: No, there it's still presented in the quotation marks of theater. I don't think of androgyny as some kind of sexy theatricality. It's an everyday way of being human, in which one has more options. Of course, men would escape from certain traps, but it's not the liberation of men that I care about mainly.

OLD ORTLEB: Let *them* eat cake.

SUSAN SONTAG: To depolarize the sexes would be more advantageous for women. Men have, in fact, something to lose—a monopoly of many kinds of power and self-confidence. China is a country which has a strongly androgynous style.

OLD ORTLEB: Now there's a forward-thinking country if there ever was one.

SUSAN SONTAG: You don't feel much difference in the way men and women come on. Women look at you with a very level gaze. They're doing the same jobs as men and they don't go through the make-up and preening thing that that has traditionally been thought part of feminine "nature." Obviously, the Chinese use androgyny for a different purpose to build something else. It's a culture which Americans and Europeans find excessively, unbelievably puritanical. Their androgyny is not leading toward sexual liberation, in our sense. But it's still a very creative, not to mention revolutionary, development—and indispensable for changing the situation of women.

OLD ORTLEB: Yes, totalitarianism has always been good for women. There is nothing more liberating than a level gaze in a androgynous totalitarian society.

YOUNG ORTLEB: In going through your essays one finds a number of your ideas coming together.

In one instance, you turn on to John Cage's idea of errorless behavior. In the essay "The Pornographic Imagination," what you seem to like is that pornography often gives one a sense that one can make a sexual connection with anyone, and then you have this concept of androgyny. Do you see this all coming together in one vision?

SUSAN SONTAG: I suppose so. But there is a larger problem which I've been thinking about since I visited China last January and February: the very role of sexuality, as such, in our lives. In our historical situation, sexual revolutions—or revolutions that center around the questioning of traditional ideas about sexual identity, sexual roles, and sexual behavior—are very creative for us. But it doesn't seem as if that revolution would be helpful to the Chinese. I suggested this at the end of the material on feminism that was published in *Partisan Review,* which was written a year before I went to China. I suggest that sex in the future will be less important if the changes we think are desirable do take place.

OLD ORTLEB: Well, that hasn't happened. Or has it?

YOUNG ORTLEB: Less orgasm oriented?

SUSAN SONTAG: Not necessarily. But less violent, less obsessional. Maybe the importance that our sexual lives has for us stems from the fact that this is the activity into which people who live in capitalist societies can put the most extreme emphasis on selfishness and on individuality—for better or worse.

OLD ORTLEB: Yeah, sex is the opiate of the people.

SUSAN SONTAG: That's where we can advance. De-emphasizing sex doesn't mean having less sex; it means not assuming that one's sexual activities are the main motors of one's life. We take it for granted that they are. The Chinese don't. And I think that their sober, monogamous society shows that our hectic sexuality is learned; it's a cultural convention. It's not so much that all people have these huge amounts of sexual energy, but that we—in our society—make a surplus investment of energy in sex, perhaps because we can't put our energy creatively into many other activities. If we develop a more communitarian, less competitive society into which we would want to put large amounts of our energies, sexuality would have to lose some of the ideological importance it has for us now.

OLD ORTLEB: Well, that's a mouthful. Sounds like a place I'd like to visit but I wouldn't want to live there.

SUSAN SONTAG: It would be less burdened with illusory "values"; it would not, by reaction, be so intimately connected with sadomasochistic provocations.

OLD ORTLEB: (*Looking at audience.*) Sell your stock in leather.

SUSAN SONTAG: Our total sexual activity wouldn't have to diminish, but sexuality as such would no longer have the responsibility of being our theater of struggle and freedom.

YOUNG ORTLEB: The persona in "Debriefing" says, "Lately, my sexual life has become very pure. I don't want it to be like a dirty movie. (Having liked a lot of dirty movies, I don't want it to be like that.) let's lie down together, love, and hold each other."

SUSAN SONTAG: You don't miss a thing do you?

OLD ORTLEB: Oh, the best is yet to come.

YOUNG ORTLEB: Is that autobiographical too?

SUSAN SONTAG: No.

OLD ORTLEB: Four Pinocchios.

YOUNG ORTLEB: Well, how do you feel about pornography now?

SUSAN SONTAG: Pornography is both liberating and terrifying, as I wrote in that essay. It's like science fiction—a kind of positive nightmare for people, and just as unrealistic and usually mechanistic. I wouldn't write "The Pornographic

Imagination" now in the same way as I did in 1965. Then I was dealing with a situation in which pornography was a civil liberties issue. It still is, because of the Supreme Court decision and because of the character of the Nixon administration. Nevertheless, a lot has happened since then. Pornography has become a big business; the esoteric literary works I was talking about are for sale at the corner drugstore; and half of the movie theaters in big cities are into hard-core. There has always been something very anti-sexual about pornography (I talk about that in the essay), and most pornographic works degrade and exploit women. It's like drugs. Our awareness of what drugs are as a big business involving the Mafia, and what drugs are as a spoiler of people's heads, is much more realistic now than in the 1960s.

YOUNG ORTLEB: Is there a contradiction of terms in the phrase "feminist pornographic imagination"? Could there ever be such a thing?

OLD ORTLEB: You are asking for trouble.

SUSAN SONTAG: I hope women will learn to feel freer about their own erotic fantasies. Most erotic fantasies are from the point of view of men. Four or five years ago Kenneth Tynan had a book project. He asked twenty English and American writers to contribute their favorite jerk-off fantasy. Everybody's name was to be on the cover but none of the entries would be signed. When he asked me to be one of the twenty, I said that didn't think I could. I doubted that I could actually write it down. And then he told me that most of the women writers he had asked to contribute had refused in much the same shy terms, while all of the men he had asked had accepted. I was really upset then, because I had thought I was confessing to a quite personal, individual inhibition. What he told me made it clear that I was simply reacting like most middle-class women writers. Women don't have the same freedom to have a sexual imagination, and to have it in public. Norman Mailer can go on broadcasting his vulgar sexual fantasies and feel quite pleased with himself, because he's a man.

OLD ORTLEB: Vulgar, nasty Norman!

SUSAN SONTAG: But most women feel, consciously or unconsciously, degraded by their own sexual fantasies. Elizabeth Hardwick put this very well in a story—it appeared in the tenth anniversary issue of *The New York Review of Books*—about being a woman and a writer. A man can fantasize in public about girls—or boys, now. That's part of the whole tradition of literature. But a woman writer who would talk in the same predatory way about the male sexual object, and how she lusts after him—"his smooth hair, the hint of coquetry in the cruel charm of his glance"—seems silly to us.

OLD ORTLEB: Nothing hotter than the coquetry of a male glance.

SUSAN SONTAG: Women writers have been notoriously prudish about their sexual fantasies. Though a spate of new confessional novels has appeared in the last year or so, it's still hard to imagine a woman Burroughs, for instance. We're still a long way from being able to write with that freedom.

YOUNG ORTLEB: Is that in your program for the next ten years?

SUSAN SONTAG: I haven't got any program. I'm just trying to stay busy being born.

YOUNG ORTLEB: In "Debriefing," the persona says that "although none of the rules for becoming more alive are valid, it's healthy to keep on formulating them." Is that very autobiographical?

SUSAN SONTAG: "Rules" suggests something confining. I mean rules in another sense—goals. The ones that create dissatisfaction. Our experience is always far more complicated than we are willing to acknowledge. There's a terrible temptation to try and simplify it. That's most of what people are doing in their heads, getting one way of understanding their experience and hanging on to that for dear life. I'm trying to make my understanding adequate to my experience. Since I learn things through writing that probably would never have come to consciousness otherwise, I want to go on writing.

YOUNG ORTLEB: The persona says, "I'm happy when I dance." Is that autobiographical?

SUSAN SONTAG: Yes.

YOUNG ORTLEB: Do you dance much?

SUSAN SONTAG: Yes. It's the opposite of what writing means. Having goals, pledging yourself to discomfort in the hope of saving your soul, has no meaning when you're out there on the floor. Thank God for dancing. (*That part of the stage goes black.*)

OLD ORTLEB: (*Holding up the magazine.*) When I finished that interview, I thought that anything was possible for me in New York. When she said," You don't miss a thing," I thought I had received the blessing of the reigning Queen of Intellectual Bohemia. I hoped it wasn't the last time I saw her. It wasn't.

Sadly, the Sontag issue was the final issue of *Out*, which only lasted for two issues.

Two years after *Out* disappeared. I still had the magazine bug and I was young enough and naïve enough about business to try and start another gay magazine. With a small group of people, I launched a gay literary magazine called *Christopher Street*. We wanted it to be a gay version of *The New Yorker*. I was told that when Gore Vidal heard that, he asked, "Well, then, what then is *The New Yorker*?" The launch was exciting and nerve-wracking. For a number of years, *Christopher Street* was the hub of gay literary culture, such as it was. We published all kinds of non-fiction, fiction, poetry, photography and interviews with established gay luminaries and future ones. Andrew Holleran, Fran Lebowitz, and Larry Kramer all graced our pages. We published a piece by Randy Shilts on Harvey Milk that eventually evolved into his book, *The Mayor of Castro Street*. We also made a stab at publishing cartoons. We were the first publication to publish the cartoons by *The New Yorker*'s Roz Chast. For a few golden years I was at the center of something special. It was the kind of publication I would have wanted to be published in. Actually, it was the only kind of publication I could have been published in. Now I was running the show. I even wrote the lines for many of the cartoons which tried to capture the gay urban zeitgeist. Like I say, we wanted to be the gay *New Yorker*.

Two years after I interviewed Sontag, she had a close call with death in the form of breast cancer. Her thinking about her encounter with cancer is what inspired her famous book, *Illness as Metaphor*. She got her cancer just about the time I was launching *Christopher Street*.

I never really expected our paths to cross again, but in the late 70s, after she had survived her cancer scare, I got a call from a friend late one afternoon. He said, "I'd like you to come over to my place for a bite. Susan Sontag is coming. It will be just the three of us."

I said some version of "Are you fucking kidding me?" and probably immediately wondered what to wear. I was at his place within an hour. He lived in some rundown building in Hell's Kitchen. When I got there, the minute he opened the door, I could see the Queen herself sitting at the kitchen table. As I struggle to recreate the moment in my mind, the thing I can see most clearly is a kind of light emanating from her face. That iconic face that was a gift from God. It was surreal. I floated in.

My friend, whose income was always a source of great mystery, had outdone himself in buying all kinds of food from Zabar's and many bottles of wine. I thought, this is going to be a serious party. My life will never get any better than this night. But now comes the bad news. I blame it on an eventful life that has been crammed with details in a memory that can only perform a kind of triage. All I can tell you about that night is that it's now a beautiful blur. It began happy and it ended happy nine hours later when we greeted the dawn of the rooftop of my friend's building with Susan Sontag. I can also tell you that I felt the kind of bond with her that one feels when they spend that much quality time with someone. I can also tell you that Susan Sontag likes to eat food, I mean, really likes to eat food. We learned more about that issue years later. I can also tell you that I loved the sound of her voice. It is a good guess that we talked about literature, literary politics in general and sexual politics in particular, because my friend had worked as a political consultant and eventually wrote for *The Nation* and he had the habit of mixing his leftist politics with his emerging militant gay identity. He may have fancied himself a gay Herbert Marcuse. My friend was one of Manhattan leftists who seemed to be able to spend many nights at the celebrity hotspot Elaine's, without having to pick up a check. He was an honest name-dropper. He really knew the names he dropped. He once invited me to brunch with Nat Hentoff and Pete Hamill. He ended up managing Bella Abzug's failed Senate campaign. It didn't surprise me when I saw both him and Susan Sontag doing cameos in Woody Allen's film *Zelig*.

Two things surprised me at the little affair. Throughout the course of the evening, Sontag smoked both dope and cigarettes. I was amazed that someone who had survived cancer would do that. The other thing I never forgot was that even though the night couldn't have been more exciting, there was moment when I must have said something that rubbed Susan the wrong way, and she must have bristled and it must have scared me enough to make a mental note to be very careful in the future because she was somewhat thin-skinned. I guess it is not something I expected from someone who is considered an intellectual and a cultural force of nature. It turned out to be a foreshadowing of revelations to come.

Even though that friend ended up hating me publicly years later for something I'll discuss shortly, I will always be grateful to him for that night with Susan Sontag that he shared with me. I'm sure all over America there are budding writers and intellectuals who dream of moving to New York City and having a literary salon night like that with someone like Susan Sontag. Well, maybe nobody has that dream anymore, or even the money to move to Manhattan.

That evening must have been a great escape from my constant anxiety about keeping my magazine in business. From the moment we published our first issue in 1976, *Christopher Street* was always on the brink of going out of business. Even though it became one of the most important cultural institutions in the gay community, there was not enough of a readership or advertising base for it to thrive. Every day it seemed less likely the publication would survive. I spent many a sleepless night trying to figure out what to do.

In late 1980, when we were hanging by a thread, I made a counterintuitive decision to start a gay newspaper to save the gay magazine. Sounds crazy, right? Back then, there were more than a few people who would have agreed with you. I hoped that by publishing a biweekly newspaper we would be able to build a bigger audience and procure more advertising from gay businesses in New York City. Inspired by one of my favorite songs, "Native New Yorker," we called it *New York Native*. It all happened so fast that I didn't even have a clue what we would put in the first issue. A man named Ronald Crumply solved that, when, while we were putting the first issue together, he entered a gay bar in Greenwich Village with a gun and killed two people and injured six. That anti-gay murder spree was the cover of our first issue with the headline, "I would have gotten more if I could," which were the words he had reportedly said to the police when he was apprehended. I ended up writing one of the major stories in the issue about the killings. I also reported on a memorial and protest that was held the night after the killings in the Village. Before the protest I went down to NYU to listen to a talk by, of all people, Michel Foucault. After his talk, many of the attendees, and Michel Foucault himself, took part in the memorial march for the men who had been murdered. I saw Susan Sontag in the audience but didn't have a chance to talk to her and I don't think she joined the march. It was the last time I saw her until sometime in 1987 or 1988.

Being the publisher and editor-in-chief of any newspaper means constantly fretting about where the next big story is going to come from and what's going to be on the cover, but I need not have worried, for within months my young newspaper would be at the center of a dark and epic story that would be the gift from Hell that never stopped giving.

In the spring of 1981, I had heard rumors that gay men who had been to the Saint Marks Baths on the Lower East Side had been coming down with a strange illness. I asked Lawrence Mass, a gay doctor, to look into it. He reported in *New York Native* that when he called the CDC, he was told that the rumors were unfounded. Those rumors turned out *not* to be unfounded on July 3 when *The New York Times* reported that a number of gay men had been coming down with a strange pneumonia. I literally started shaking uncontrollably after I read that story.

In the ensuing days and weeks, I struggled to get a grip on the emerging amorphous facts about the mysterious new disease while grappling with the state of severe anxiety that the terrifying news had aroused in me and the rest of the community.

Everyone not in a state of denial wondered how bad it was going to get.

I sensed that what was happening was going to be a huge event that would determine my newspaper's place in history. I tried to remain optimistic. I told myself that in an age of scientific and technological genius and daily miracles surely the cause would be found and a cure would follow. Wasn't that how science operated?

From 1981 to early in 1983, every kind of scientific hypothesis about the cause of what became known as AIDS was covered in my newspaper. As a publisher eager to know every possibility and to share all emerging information with the readers of *New York Native*, I was willing to listen to anyone who had an idea. I was constantly on the phone with doctors, scientists, and other members of the media.

During the first two years of the epidemic, I was generally trustful of the government scientists at the CDC. They seemed sincere and decent. Emphasis on "seemed." The scientists I talked to did not *seem* particularly anti-gay, although disconcerting AIDS jokes were beginning to circulate even among scientists and doctors. Like, "What does 'Gay' stand for? Got AIDS yet?"

Our reporting on the epidemic took more and more space in *New York Native* and there were many gay people who wanted us to downplay the issue because it was bad for the image of the community. One prominent gay businessman who was our largest advertiser said he would stop advertising in *New York Native* if we didn't stop making AIDS our constant cover story.

I dug my heels in. I felt it was *New York Native's* responsibility to be the paper of record on AIDS. We would do what *The New York Times* and the rest of the media was failing to do. As a result of our commitment, David Black wrote an article in *Rolling Stone* in which he said *New York Native* deserved a Pulitzer Prize for its reporting. And Randy Shilts praised our pioneering and thorough reporting on AIDS in his book *And the Band Played On*. Me and my newspaper were the subject of a major profile in *Rolling Stone* by Katie Leishman. It was appropriately titled "The Outsider."

In March of 1983, we published what would turn out to be the most consequential and talked-about pieces in *New York Native's* history. At 5,000 words, it was also the longest. The title was "1,112 and Counting," and it was written by screenwriter and novelist Larry Kramer. The 1,112, of course, was the number of Americans who had died from AIDS at that point. It was a call to arms about the seriousness of the epidemic and many consider it the article that helped launch the AIDS activist movement. For better or worse.

Like all of Kramer's articles, he pleaded with gay men to get angry. He wrote, "If this doesn't scare the shit out of you, we're in real trouble. If this article doesn't rouse you to anger, fury, rage, and action, gay men may have no future on earth. Our continued existence depends on just how angry you can get."

Shortly after we published the piece, I received a phone call from John Berendt, a magazine editor who, years later, wrote the bestselling book, *Midnight in the Garden of Good and Evil*. Berendt was intrigued by an article he read about a young scientist, Jane Teas, who suggested that AIDS was caused by African Swine Fever Virus, a pig virus that had spread from Africa to Haiti, the Dominican Republic, Brazil, and Cuba in the years leading up to the AIDS epidemic. The virus caused a spectrum of AIDS-like illnesses in pigs. Teas suggested that it had spread to humans as many pig illnesses do. It was an idea totally based on epidemiological common sense. It was not a stretch. The idea was so reasonable that I asked our reporter, Dr. James D'Eramo, to go to Boston to interview Teas. When he got back and briefed me on the interview, I was so impressed that I put "Is It African Swine Fever?" on the cover of the next issue of *New York Native*.

We devoted many issues of *New York Native* to the African Swine Fever story and the attempts by Jane Teas to get her hypothesis tested. There was a great deal of hostile resistance at the CDC and the United States Department of Agriculture to her idea, which puzzled me. Why was there such a rush to judgment? There were so many similarities between AIDS and African Swine Fever that frankly, it seemed like the very best hypothesis. I got in touch with an insider at the United States Department of Agriculture and he agreed it was a plausible theory. We found a retired expert on African Swine Fever who had worked on the virus all his professional life and he wrote a letter in support of Teas.

Jane Teas eventually was able to test the blood of a group of AIDS patients for African Swine Fever. A significant number of the AIDS patients were positive for African Swine Fever Virus, but the Centers for Disease Control and the USDA did everything they could to discredit her findings. You can read about all the twists and turns of her struggle in my history of *New York Native*.

As we all know, the government eventually declared a retrovirus subsequently called HIV the cause of AIDS. While this was a great relief for the whole world, for my newspaper the news was received with a grain of salt because we knew a great deal about the previous work of the scientists who were behind the so-called discovery, and they were questionable characters, most specifically Robert Gallo, someone I have called the Richard Nixon of science, though these days I would probably call him the Donald Trump of science.

New York Native was the first newspaper to make Robert Gallo's science and character a major issue. A gay scientist who was in Boston at a luncheon with Gallo reported to us that Gallo referred to gay people as "homos." One of the leading AIDS doctors in Manhattan told me that scientists in Europe considered him a crook. The more I learned about Gallo and his history of stealing scientific discoveries and playing fast and loose with the truth in science, the less I trusted the whole heavy-handed HIV story of AIDS, especially in light of the very political way the CDC and USDA had handled the African Swine Fever issue.

When we first learned that Gallo's laboratory was falsifying all kinds of data and playing games with the retrovirus that was eventually declared the cause of AIDS, I did an explosive cover with the headline that said, "Should Gallo Be in Jail?" I had a heated conversation with Gallo after that came out and became more convinced that something was wrong with him. One prominent gay attorney I knew asked to have a drink with me the day that issue came out. When I arrived at the bar, he startled me when he immediately pulled the Gallo issue of *New York Native* out of his briefcase and said in a haughty tone of voice, "You must stop doing this." Channeling Tina Turner, my response was, "I'm just getting started." That was an early sign that the gay community didn't want to be exposed to any journalism about the epidemic that challenged the AIDS establishment. A worrisome, obsequious, and abject state of mind had overtaken the gay community. It paved the way for what I would eventually call a lemming culture of Useful AIDS Idiots.

The insider I was in touch with at the high-security USDA research facilities on Plum Island was, at the time, probably the world's most accomplished African Swine Fever scientist. He became my Deep Throat at the USDA. He privately took issue with what we were being told by the authorities about African Swine Fever. His boss, the Director of the Plum Island facility that did research on African Swine Fever, crankily insisted that AIDS and African Swine Fever were not in any way similar. That was a total lie. Several years later, a textbook came out which said in its first paragraph that African Swine Fever could be considered the AIDS of pigs. Perhaps the most explosive thing we ever published was a story noting that we had received word from inside the USDA that some pigs in New Jersey and

New York had tested positive for African Swine Fever.

When Jane Teas and a colleague finally performed experiments and found that a significant number of AIDS patients were infected with African Swine Fever, Robert Gallo invited the gay scientist who had collaborated with her to make a presentation of their research in Gallo's lab. He was cordially received by Gallo and his staff. Gallo even took him out to dinner. Gallo told the gay scientist that after he saw what they had done he understood why they thought ASFV was the cause, but nothing came of it. Well, not exactly nothing. In a matter of months, Gallo's lab claimed to have discovered a new DNA virus in AIDS and Chronic Fatigue Syndrome patients. That virus eventually was called Human Herpes Virus 6. The gay collaborator who worked with Teas suspected that Gallo had done something he had done with HIV, which is rename African Swine Fever Virus. This kind of game is much easier to play in science than most people realize.

Gallo's HHV-6 discovery would always have two dark clouds of suspicion above it. In addition to the suspicion that Gallo had just stolen the work of Jane Teas and her colleague, and renamed their DNA virus, there was the potentially explosive realization among some that the new DNA virus, HHV-6, was the real cause of AIDS and Chronic Fatigue

Syndrome. That would mean HIV was a big mistake, potentially a huge embarrassment to the CDC and growing AIDS establishment. Early on, HIV had become an article of faith. To question it was to question the existence of God. Thanks to AIDS, science had morphed into religion.

If HHV-6 had been recognized as the real cause of both AIDS and Chronic Fatigue Syndrome, that would have indicated that they were part of one epidemic that was a spectrum of illnesses. There could possibly be many more immunological illnesses on that HHV-6 spectrum. It would also mean that—hold your breath--AIDS was not, strictly speaking, a sexually transmitted disease. Yes, you heard that correctly. *Not* a sexually transmitted disease. You can breathe now.

We published many more eye-opening stories that put the credibility of the CDC in doubt. I was in touch with a gay man who eventually worked in the Director's office at the CDC. He leaked the troubling news that the CDC was manipulating the results of HIV tests. He informed us that when the CDC was determining the dividing line between a positive and a negative result for HIV, if a gay man and a straight man had the same borderline reading, the gay man would be marked as positive and the straight man would be a negative. You could call it diagnosis by risk group.

For the first couple years of the epidemic, the CDC loved *New York Native* because we basically reported whatever information they were sharing with the public. We were getting *their word* out to the gay community. But as I started to wonder about the honesty and integrity of both the CDC and the USDA, our reporting became less like stenography and more skeptical and investigative. We were beginning to look beneath the masks of the epidemic and those institutions didn't like that. James Curran, the top CDC AIDS researcher, started getting testy with me on the phone and asked sarcastically if I thought he was being homophobic. And then he just didn't return my phone calls, which, generally speaking, is how doctors and scientists can control the flow of information. If you don't play ball, you don't get information. That's why you will find that most scientific and medical reporters are puppets and patsies. There are no cold-blooded science and medicine reporters. Basically, they all suck.

Because we couldn't fight City Hall on the issue of African Swine Fever, we decided to do as much investigative reporting on HHV-6 as we could, which, as I have pointed out, linked AIDS and Chronic Fatigue Syndrome and many other epidemics. If it could be established that HHV-6 was the real cause of both AIDS and Chronic Fatigue Syndrome, the issues of whether HHV-6 really was African Swine Fever Virus and credit for the discovery of the real cause of AIDS had been stolen from Jane Teas could be settled later.

As I look back, the most explosive story we ever published was one I published in 1986 by a reporter named Ann Fettner. She located a man who was doing AIDS epidemiology work for the CDC in Florida and what he said about the AIDS researchers in Atlanta was disturbing, to put it mildly. He said that his bosses at the CDC were basically falsifying the data about AIDS that was coming out of Florida. They blamed him for not asking patients the right questions when his data showed that people in Florida who were getting AIDS didn't fit into the CDC's AIDS behavioral risk groups. His data supported the notion that AIDS was not limited to the so-called risk groups and it was not, strictly speaking, a sexually transmitted disease predominantly confined to the gay community. Anything that didn't support the STD hypothesis was politically incorrect. It also meant that AIDS was a far bigger epidemic than anyone thought. The Florida CDC employee told Fettner that 90% of what was going on at the CDC around AIDS was just public relations. He said that the CDC researchers involved in AIDS were basically liars and clueless kids who had just gotten out of medical school. His bosses were so committed to covering up what was going on that, in retrospect, it seems clear that far more was known at the CDC about the true nature of the epidemic *right from the beginning*. Had those cases that conflicted with the party line been brought to the public's attention, we might now be talking about a completely different epidemic and a different cause from HIV. Chronic Fatigue Syndrome would not still be a so-called mystery.

That Florida CDC employee, by the way, was punished for speaking up by being transferred. It was one of the early signs of how dissent was going to be handled in the emerging dark and deceitful empire of AIDS research. It should have been clear back then that AIDS was AIDSgate.

Those cases that were covered up in Florida might have made it difficult for the CDC to create a wall of apartheid between AIDS and Chronic Fatigue Syndrome that stands to this very day.

One of the most interesting developments we reported on was a trip Jane Teas made to an area of Florida that had a lot of AIDS cases. What she also found in the same area was a lot of sick pigs, which helped support her notion that the whole epidemic originated in sick pigs. The information could have blown the AIDS paradigm to smithereens. But the CDC's HIV STD dogma was quickly becoming the conventional wisdom.

We also published an underappreciated story by freelance reporter who had gone to Haiti to do a story on AIDS and discovered that in an area where there was an epidemic of African Swine Fever there were a number of mysterious human deaths.

It all got curiouser and curiouser. We also reported on a major scandal that involved AIDS experiments being sabotaged and tampered with at the CDC. It also appeared that evidence was being destroyed. Something was definitely rotten in Denmark, but the mainstream media was looking the other way.

One of the most important stories I reported on myself was about a doctor in Atlanta, the same city in which the CDC is located. That doctor was seeing heterosexual people with the malady that eventually became known as Chronic Fatigue Syndrome at the same time as the so-called AIDS cases were first being identified. It is possible that those cases which also involved immune dysfunction could have been the Patient Zeros of the real AIDS epidemic. But the CDC didn't include the Chronic Fatigue Syndrome patients in Atlanta in their AIDS cases. They deliberately looked the other way. After all, they were heterosexuals.

All of this was happening, by the way, at the same time that William F. Buckley said on his PBS show *Firing Line*, that "Everyone detected with AIDS should be tattooed in the upper forearm to protect common-needle users, and on the buttocks, to protect the victimization of other homosexuals." He would never dare suggest that for white heterosexuals with Chronic Fatigue Syndrome.

In June of 1987, we introduced our readers to the thinking of Peter Duesberg. He was a celebrated retrovirologist who was expected to eventually win a Nobel Prize. He had a rotating grant from NIH that was sometimes referred to as a "genius grant." In a publication called *Cancer Research*, he published a paper arguing that there was no way that HIV could be the cause of AIDS. As you can imagine, his dissent—or whistleblowing—set the AIDS establishment's hair on fire. The AIDS establishment was quickly becoming the HIV establishment and didn't want to turn back. Whistleblowers, critics, and dissenters had to be ignored or destroyed. Duesberg ultimately did not have his NIH grant renewed and was generally smeared in the media as a threat to public health. Even *The New Yorker* ultimately went after him.

In the same month I made the case in an editorial that one could only conclude from the reporting in *New York Native* that the emerging epidemic of Chronic Fatigue Syndrome was actually the other face of the AIDS epidemic, and that the virus that linked the two epidemics and made them one variable epidemic was Human Herpes Virus 6, the virus that the colleague of Jane Teas thought Gallo had stolen credit for discovering by renaming African Swine Fever Virus.

In October of 1987, we began to publish a series of investigative articles by John Lauritsen that presented a sinister picture of the so-called science that was conducted to support the use of AZT in AIDS patients. In several articles he made the compelling case that much of the AZT research was fudged and the drug was killing patients. The treatment was worse than the disease.

In November of that year, I got a call from someone in the Reagan White House because there was concern that HIV was not really the cause of AIDS. They wanted to have a White House meeting at which Peter Duesberg could make his case that HIV was a big mistake. Unfortunately, the man who turned out to be the most powerful scientist in AIDS, someone who could be called the puppet master or Czar of both AIDS and Chronic Fatigue Syndrome scientific fraud, Anthony Fauci, succeeded in getting the meeting cancelled. Fauci was an expert at manipulating politicians and the media through browbeating and veiled threats. What did the White House know about science? How dare they stick their nose into Fauci's growing public health empire. The White House quickly got religion about HIV.

Around that time, I got wind of the fact that Susan Sontag was working on a book about AIDS. It took some doing, but I was able to reach her at the place she had moved to in SoHo. I was thrilled when she agreed to see me, and I nervously prepared to brief her on everything we had been reporting on. I thought that Susan would be the conduit to the mainstream media and the New York intelligentsia for of our little newspaper's investigative reporting. I thought for sure she would recognize that the basic premises of the government scientists working on AIDS were questionable at best.

As I recall the meeting, which I think lasted for a couple of hours, she couldn't have been nicer. As I outlined the basic conclusions of our first six years of reporting on the epidemic, she seemed very interested in what I had to say. I remember one moment when we were talking about some technical medical issue, and she got up to find a very big medical textbook. In retrospect, it felt like she was trying—in a dramatic manner—to give me the impression that she really knew her way around science. In the years that followed, whenever I remember her with that big medical textbook, it made me think of Lily Tomlin doing Edith Ann in the big rocking chair. I had no reason to think that the meeting was for naught. The most memorable moment occurred at my departure. She hugged me and said, "You've always been very real to me."

"You've always been very real to me?" It sounded good, but I remember saying to myself, "What the fuck does that mean?" And, "Why wouldn't I be very real to you?" Were most of the people in her life from another planet? Were they all phonies? It turned out that Susan herself was from another planet.

It would be at least a year before her *AIDS and Its Metaphors* came out and, the day it did, I anxiously rushed to the bookstore and immediately devoured the book. Well, the only way I can describe my reaction to *AIDS and Its Metaphors* is to tell you about a Fourth of July experience I had when I was a kid. My family had moved to a state that had rather loose laws about fireworks, and somehow all the kids on our block were allowed to set firecrackers off. They were not cherry bombs. They were small but they were not harmless. I was having fun lighting them and throwing them in the air until I didn't throw one fast enough and it blew up in my hand. No, I didn't lose a finger, but a flash of terror went through my mind that I did. My hand was slightly burned and had turned black. My ears would not stop ringing, and I felt a kind of shock throughout my whole body. I couldn't believe that such a thing had happened to me.

That's how I felt when it was clear to me that Susan had attacked me and my newspaper without even naming me or my newspaper. I felt the kind of shock and rage that induces tears. I could not believe it. My newspaper was operating on a shoestring, taking on the growing AIDS establishment, doing serious investigative reporting and breaking one major story after another that made us the virtual Woodward and Bernstein operation of the AIDS epidemic, and this woman that I had adored and looked up to decided to shit all over our unrelenting coverage of AIDS in a pretentious, pedantic little book.

I know I had only spent time with her on three occasions, but it was meaningful time. Maybe I wasn't someone special in her life, but I thought that to some degree we were friends, that she at least respected me. That she would never do anything gratuitously to hurt me or my newspaper. To this day, that pain is still, as she would say, very real to me.

I found her number and left an angry message on her answering machine. Somehow, I knew I would never hear from her again, and I didn't.

It's been over thirty years since *AIDS and Its Metaphors* came out, so I have had a lot of time to let my thoughts about her and her book marinate.

(*Looking at audience.*) Nobody called me up to commiserate. That was because she didn't say my name or *New York Native* in the book, but *I knew*. And it was sneaky. She knew *exactly* what she was doing.

For me it was just the beginning of me seeing the dark, unexpected side of Susan Sontag.

(*Looking over at Susan.*) Susan, I never got a chance to tell you what I thought of *AIDS and Its Metaphors*. So here goes.

You wrote that you wanted basically "to calm the imagination not to incite it."[1] That is a pretty good way to describe some forms of public health propaganda, which is essentially what *AIDS and Its Metaphors* is. Don't scare the horses. Scare the gays.

You urged people to get competent treatment, but you avoided the question of whether the science of AIDS was competent and honest. I had warned you that *it was not*. If you had taken the reporting of my newspaper seriously, your message would have been totally different.

You thought that if we could correct the way we talk about AIDS, we could remove the stigma. But it was a matter of how the Centers for Disease Control talked about AIDS, not the dummies you were clearly directing your smarter-than-thou message.

What you didn't grasp is the stigmatizing power of the paradigm created by fraudulent science. And you didn't perceive what an evil existential paradigm gay people were already trapped in even before the descent of the CDC's gerrymandered AIDS paradigm. Gay people were already life unworthy of life when the CDC's epidemiology descended. You helped push them deeper into the CDC's quicksand.

You thought you had helped lift the stigma of cancer in your previous book, *Illness as Metaphor*. But *AIDS and Its Metaphors* did nothing but help the CDC carve its stigmatizing and false epidemiology into stone.

Yes, you said that AIDS has a single cause, but you didn't acknowledge any doubts that the official cause was based on data that was not trustworthy and was skewed by homophobia, racism and corrupt power politics. You ignored all the signs of scientific fraud my newspaper had uncovered.

Your understanding of AIDS seemed to rely heavily on Manhattan's Bible, *The New York Times*. You were clueless about the old-boy-network politics of their scientific reporting, that the *Times*'s lead AIDS reporter had worked for the CDC. You were clearly unaware that science and medical reporting at *The New York Times* was more like agitprop than investigative reporting.

The only serious, independent, skeptical, critical, reporting was being done by my newspaper, *New*

York Native, and I had brought it to you on a silver platter.

You used expressions like "the construction of the illness,"[2] but you never seriously questioned *who or what* was doing the constructing. I could name the names. I have named the names. The first signs that homophobia and racism were undergirding the pseudoscience and gerrymandered epidemiology were already visible when I met with you.

Every time you accepted the premise that AIDS was a sexually transmitted disease, you served the purpose of all Useful AIDS Idiots who act as conveyor belts for the CDC's dogmatic narrative.

You said that most people outside of Africa know how they got it.[3] Well, they *think* they know how they got it. The CDC and *The New York Times* told them how they got it. And Useful AIDS Idiots told them how they got it. But the job of intellectuals and serious newspapers is to audit that dogma, to investigate that dogma, to look behind the rigid pronouncements. What you did in *AIDS and Its Metaphors* is to play word games around the edges to the real issue and act like, for the most part, the fundamentals of AIDS consisted of settled science. As though there were no credibility gaps. Hey Susan, remember the credibility gaps of the Vietnam War? Remember what Hannah Arendt wrote about them?

You know Susan, it turned out that you worshipped Hannah Arendt. AIDS desperately needed a Hannah Arendt. Instead it got a Susan Sontag.

You wrote that the majority of cases were among members of "a risk group, a community of pariahs."[4] Well Susan, who established those pariah risk groups? Where were the challenging second opinions?

You note that the disease "isolates the ill and exposes them to harassment and persecution."[5] True enough, Susan, but who created that paradigm that left them in that precarious position? If you had looked closer, Susan, you would have seen that it was the usual suspects. Epidemiology is political, Susan.

You wrote, "The unsafe behavior that produces AIDS is judged to be more than just weakness. It is indulgence, delinquency—addictions to chemicals that are illegal and to sex regarded as deviant."[6] It didn't take AIDS to impose that kind of stigmatizing discourse about gay people. Gay people were associated with disease even before this disease occurred. And by the way, any talk of behavior producing AIDS makes you a four-star Useful AIDS Idiot. It was the *pseudoscientific behavior* that produced the AIDS paradigm you should have been focused on. Homophobic behavior. Racist behavior.

Susan, did it ever occur to you that the dogma that AIDS was essentially a reflection of cognitive bias and failed epidemiological due diligence? Was that a bridge too far?

Yes, Susan, you are correct when you wrote, "An infectious disease whose principle means of transmission is sexual necessarily puts at greater risk those who are sexually more active—and is easy to view as a punishment for that activity."[7] But no Susan, not if the epidemiology is a crock. You should have been focused on the principle transmission vehicles of the AIDS paradigm and treacherous AIDS fraud: you and Useful AIDS Idiots like yourself.

You wrote, "Getting the disease through a sexual practice is thought to be more willful, therefore deserves more blame."[8] Thought by whom, Susan? You? Your scientist friends at Harvard? Where do you place scientific fraud on the willfulness and blame scale?

It was pure poetry when you wrote the words, "Promiscuous homosexual men practicing their vehement customs."[9] Promiscuous homosexual men practicing their vehement sexual customs? I can imagine the moralizing thrill going up your leg when you hit upon the word "vehement." More was going on here than meets the eye, I think, Susan.

You wrote, "Infectious diseases to which sexual fault is attached always inspires fear of easy contagion and bizarre fantasies of transmission by nonveneral means in public places."[10] Bizarre? Always inspires? To suggest that a better understanding of the epidemiological pattern actually suggested nonveneral transmission is a bizarre fantasy? You were kind of cutting off free thought at the pass, don't you think Susan? Anyone who challenged the paradigm could be marginalized as bizarre. Maybe even crazy. Maybe even deplorable.

What you and all Useful AIDS Idiots did was make it difficult to see what ultimately turned out to be the real epidemic. You made the fake epidemic look sane and the real epidemic look crazy. This is how the culture of what I now call Manhattan Cosmopolitan Cliquishness operates. Anything your tribe doesn't believe is beyond the pale, alternative facts, fake news. All your intellectual opponents were bizarre fantasizers. Sanity could only be found in the pages of *The New York Times*, *The New Yorker*, or *The New York Review of Books*.

I assume you considered the investigative reporting of my little gay newspaper to be bizarre fantasizing. After all, most of its audience practiced "vehement sexual customs." When they weren't being purveyors of "camp."

You noted that AIDS is "not a single illness" and is "a product of definition or construction."[11] But you never really had any serious questions about the source of the definition or the construction. The questionable source was what I had travelled to SoHo to warn you about.

You acted like it was all a matter of avoiding the wrong words, the wrong metaphors, as though the real problem was the language in which the epidemic was presented and discussed. But what about the facts, the science beneath the wordplay of the narrative? What about the wordplay of the science itself? What about the wordplay of homophobia and racism that went on in the minds of the young scientists and epidemiologists who crafted the paradigm of AIDS that separated it from the Chronic Fatigue Syndrome epidemic in white heterosexuals? You were great at fancy, pedantic rhetoric, but Susan, you had real problems with reality.

What did you think my newspaper was presenting to its readers? Chopped liver?

To your credit, you accurately noted that the mortality rate of AIDS could have been an artifact that hid the possibility that the disease, whatever it really was, was not universally fatal. You noticed the way the authorities were hedging their bets. But you didn't see the extent to which the CDC was playing games with the declared facts of the epidemic and its epidemiology.

You never considered the fact that they, like the best and the brightest during the Vietnam War, were hiding the truth about the epidemic from themselves in *their* words and *their* metaphors and *their* epidemiological narrative. You never considered the possibility that the fear of the truth about AIDS and ultimately Chronic Fatigue Syndrome could be found at the very heart of the misguided science at the CDC. I tried to convince you that the whole megillah was on shaky ground. Unsuccessfully, but I tried.

You never focused on the epidemic's biggest linguistic mask of all, the term "Human Immunodeficiency Virus" or HIV. Those words were imposed on the epidemic by fiat and repeated ad nauseum. To not question those words and acknowledge the dissent and critical thinking about them was one of the most important acts of a Useful AIDS Idiot. You failed to notice that the term "Human Immunodeficiency Virus" was imposed on a virus as a kind of bum's rush to get every other explanation for the epidemic off the stage. Causation was established by the fiat of using that name for the agent only *associated* with the disease, and—if you had looked closely—not even with all cases. You failed to recognize the distinct aroma of CDC groupthink.

You and a voluntary army of Useful AIDS Idiots became the unpaid boosters of HIV propaganda.

You asserted that the predictions about AIDS "have seemed mostly an exercise in the management of public opinion."[12] You ignored our reporting and my warning that all of the so-called basic science and epidemiology coming out of the CDC was fundamentally "management of public opinion."

Like a good Manhattan liberal, you listed all the horrifying social consequences of testing positive for HIV, but once again, like a good Useful AIDS idiot, you failed to consider that the science of AIDS might be as reliable as a body count during the Vietnam war.

You wrote, "With the most up-to-date biomedical testing, it is possible to create a new class of lifetime pariahs, the future ill."[13] Susan, if you had listened to what I told you and questioned the legitimacy of the paradigm you might have been able to help liberate that class of pariahs.

One of the creepiest lines in your book was, "A predictable mix of superstition and resignation is leading some people with AIDS to refuse antiviral chemotherapy."[14] When I first read that I thought, well, fuck you Susan. You wrote that at the time when the drug AZT was being foisted—and I do mean foisted—on AIDS patients. As was detailed in the investigative reporting by John Lauritsen that we published, it was an insane drug that killed the very cells it supposedly was being used to save. AZT brought the word genocide into the AIDS conversation. You made a conscious decision to ignore all that reporting. How dare you, from your supercilious pedestal, call the critical thinking, investigative reporting and resistance to such a fraud-based toxic drug that endangered lives a predictable mix of superstition and resignation.

The poor gay men who were scared out of their wits and had to figure out so much for themselves in the face of such social and medical hostility were *predictably full of superstition and resignation*? What baloney! If more of them had resisted the medical establishment and the culture of Useful AIDS Idiots that you enabled, maybe the whole story of AIDS would have been different. And the story of Chronic Fatigue Syndrome. And your personal story.

No, there were no good treatments back then, but maybe there would have been if the epidemiology of AIDS had not been a tissue of lies and self-deceptions, just like Vietnam. You wrote, "But subjecting an emaciating body to the purification of a macrobiotic diet is about as helpful in treating AIDS as having oneself bled, the "holistic" medical treatment of choice in the era of Donne."[15] Very nice Susan. Very snarky. You totally ignored what happened when those emaciated bodies were pumped up with high doses of AZT. You ignored the fraud that was discovered in the AZT research by my reporter. The air of frankly homophobic condescension that runs throughout your piece belonged in William F. Buckley's *National Review.* Those who chose macrobiotics over AZT may actually *have* bought themselves a little more time, something you yourself eventually were not unfamiliar with.

Like some, but not all, Useful AIDS idiots, you seemed to be writing about a terrifying phenomenon that you really didn't think threatened *you* personally. How ironic, given what would happen to you fifteen years after the publication of *AIDS and Its Metaphors.*

You wrote, "AIDS is understood in a premodern way, as a disease incurred by people both as individuals and members of a risk group—that neutral sounding bureaucratic category which also revives the archaic idea of a tainted community that illness has judged."[16]

Susan, I warned you that all that malarkey about a "tainted community" was being concocted by scientists whose competence and honesty could not be trusted. They were the gang that couldn't shoot straight. They were the Keystone Cops of medical science and epidemiology.

You seemed to love the idea of thinking critically and objectively about the disease but that was not what was going on in your nasty little book. It was, however, what was going on in my little newspaper that you didn't even have the decency to name in your stealth attack.

The part of your book where you took direct aim at me and my newspaper went like this: "The subliminal connection made to notions about a primitive past and many hypotheses that have been fielded about possible transmission from animals (a disease of green monkeys? African Swine Fever?) cannot but activate a familiar set of stereotypes about animality, sexual disease and blacks."[17]

Really, Susan? African Swine Fever cannot help but activate stereotypes about blacks? The idea that a pig virus which causes an AIDS-like illness in pigs could also cause AIDS in people is inherently racist, an appeal to racist stereotypes? Is that what you were suggesting was behind our investigative reporting?

God forbid you noted for your readers that my newspaper had been catching the CDC and the Department of Agriculture in a whole series of lies.

Anyone who questions the dogma of Useful AIDS Idiots will be accused of being a deplorable or a conspiracy theorist. We know how that game works. That game has gotten even uglier since your book came out. Anyone who disagrees with anyone about anything is now either a conspiracy theorist or a denialist.

You made patronizing fun of the Russian disinformation campaign that blamed the CIA for engineering HIV, but you conveniently ignored credible reporting in *Newsday* that the CIA introduced African Swine Fever to Cuba. That wasn't fake news. But that didn't fit into your Useful AIDS Idiot sexually transmitted disease narrative.

Much of your Useful AIDS Idiot book is a kind of white heterosexual whistling in the dark, which is odd, coming from a quasi-lesbian, or whatever it is that you were, Susan.

You wrote, "At first it was assumed that AIDS must become widespread elsewhere in the same catastrophic form in which it has emerged in Africa and those who still think it will eventually happen invariably invoke the Black Death."[18] Well, not everyone, Susan. My newspaper made the case in its reporting that it had already taken on a catastrophic form in the United State, but that it was a spectrum of immunological dysfunction hidden behind the mask of Chronic Fatigue Syndrome. You knew a lot about masks Susan. You were a one-woman Halloween.

The idea that AIDS would have a global spread was not coming from a benighted idea that the epidemic was some kind of judgment from God. It was based on the common-sense analysis that assuming the epidemic in Africa couldn't happen in any form in America was a form of denial, magical racist thinking. Like most Useful AIDS Idiots, you were building the walls around the politically incorrrect thoughts about the epidemic. A typical gaslighting tactic of Useful AIDS Idiots.

Susan, no matter how much you played with words, teased out their origins, their ironies and their boneheaded misuses, you avoided the big question of whether the basic science and STD epidemiology of AIDS that you took for granted are totally bogus, as false as blaming ulcers on stress. I warned you as much as I could—in the two hours I spent with you—that it was a house of cards. I tried to prevent you from becoming a clueless parrot for the false AIDS narrative. You showed how easily intellectuals can become tony instruments of disinformation.

You were right to say that sexually transmitted diseases were traditionally "described as punishments not just of individuals but of a group."[19] But you never asked whether the CDC had turned a disease that was not technically an STD into a paradigm maintained by deception, self-deception, and propaganda.

You noted that disease could be used "didactically."[20] What the Hell did you think you were doing in your book?

You recognize disease can be used to "punish and censor."[21] But why didn't you acknowledge the CDC's role in that? That the science was fudged and disfigured into an image that could punish and censor? I'll tell you what punished and censored: *AIDS and Its Metaphors.*

Ironically, you discuss *The White Plague,* a play about an imaginary plague written by Karel Capek. You noted that in his play, "He scores didactic points by focusing not on the disease itself but the management of information about it by scientists, journalists, and politicians."[22] That is a perfect description of AIDS and unfortunately, *you* helped manage information about an epidemic of lies. You called Capek's play "A not improbable sketch of catastrophe . . . as a managed public event in modern mass society."[23] Your book helped manage the public event of AIDS. You helped sell the image of AIDS as a mostly gay sexually transmitted disease which was the nucleus of the CDC's Big Lie. You helped build the wall of apartheid between AIDS and Chronic Fatigue Syndrome and all the illnesses on the HHV-6 spectrum.

Why was it so unthinkable, so unimaginable, that the CDC and NIH got the whole thing wrong? I *mean the whole thing.* Why was it out of the question? I warned you in person not to buy their narrative, hook, line, and sinker. AIDS was a public relations facade you were not truly able or willing to look behind. Perhaps you were afraid to. Exactly what was wrong with you? You were the one who said communism is fascism with a human face. Why was it a bridge too far for you to see that HIVism was becoming fascism with a public health face? Did you not grasp how easily epidemiology can become an arm of totalitarianism?

You helped promote a *fake scapegoating* epidemic that hid the *real* catastrophic epidemic. You were clueless in your book that you were helping to hide a viral epidemic of the HHV-6 family of viruses that the CDC insisted had nothing to do with African Swine Fever. Everyone on this planet is going to have to deal with that family of viruses one way or another. You may already have.

And, *predictably*, you made fun of people who saw AIDS as a plague that threatened everyone. Yes, those people included bigots like Norman Podhoritz, Jerry Falwell, and Pat Buchanan. But the epidemic was what it was. The easy transmissibility of the real epidemic hidden beneath the Useful AIDS Idiot STD version of the epidemic was not an evil rightwing paranoid fantasy. But you bought the CDC dogma and helped them turn scientific fraud into an article of faith. You helped turn critical thinkers and investigative reporters into pariahs. You helped make it dangerous to see the truth. You helped make it dangerous to publish it.

You seemed determined to debunk any language or metaphor that creates "the sense of the omnipresence of AIDS."[24] Basically, it seems like you were trying to convince yourself and the rest of the public that you were not at risk. AIDS, the mostly gay male STD was not really something you needed to fear. You, no doubt, probably thought your own behavior protected you. You didn't have vehement customs. Boy was your own body in for a big surprise.

You wrote that "AIDS marks a turning point in current attitudes toward illness and medicine, as well as toward sexuality and toward catastrophe."[25] Yes, Susan, because you, as a Useful AIDS Idiot, helped carry that CDC water.

You assisted the CDC in delivering its propaganda loud and clear when you wrote, "Now AIDS obliges people to think of sex as having possibly, the direst of consequences: suicide or murder."[26] That sentence made you as important to the CDC's HIV/AIDS Reich as Leni Riefenstahl was to the Third Reich.

You wrote, "Fear of sexuality is the new, disease-sponsored register of the universe of fear in which everyone lives."[27] The one fear you didn't write about was the fear that all the science and epidemiology it was based on were fudged, cooked, cherry-picked, and driven by an antigay agenda that poisoned all the public health pronouncements about the epidemic.

Susan, you would have fit in perfectly in the public relations department at the CDC when you wrote, "The view that sexually transmitted diseases are not serious reached its apogee in the 1970s, which was also when many male homosexuals reconstituted themselves as something like an ethnic group, one whose distinctive folkloric custom was sexual voracity, and the institutions of urban homosexual life became a sexual delivery system of unprecedented speed, efficiency, and volume."[28] To borrow a line from Molly Ivins, I'm sure that sentence was even better in the original German.

The goofiest part of your book is the one in which you tie gay sexual appetite to the culture of capitalism. There you combine being a modern Useful AIDS Idiot with being an old fashioned Marxist-Leninist Useful Idiot. You seem to be cheering on the cultural changes that the AIDS epidemic was bringing. You seem to support the AIDS-related call for "self-management" and "self-discipline."[29] The new cosmopolitan public health Marxist nanny was pointing her puritanical finger. And meanwhile, the Rome of the HHV-6 and Chronic Fatigue Syndrome epidemic burned.

I didn't know exactly where the call for limits on "the indulgence of certain habits" was coming from when I first read your book. But now I do.

You wrote, "The response to AIDS, while in part perfectly rational, amplifies a widespread questioning that had been rising in in intensity throughout the 1970s of many of the ideals (and risks) of enlightened modernity; and the new sexual realism goes with the rediscovery of tonal music, Bouguereau, a career in investment banking and church weddings."[30] Well, Susan, you can stick your tonal music, your Bouguereau, your career in investment banking, and your church weddings where the sun don't shine because it was all based on pseudoscientific hogwash.

You wrote, "Demands are made to subject to 'tests,' to isolate the ill and those suspected of being ill or of transmitting illness, and to erect barriers against the real or imaginary contamination of foreigners."[31] Yes, Susan, but why? Because you and fellow elite opinion leaders didn't perform serious due diligence and you didn't pay attention to what was in *New York Native*. You didn't even question the legitimacy of the tests. You don't have the luxury of an excuse that nobody warned you.

Near the end of your book, after basically presenting AIDS as a gay STD, you note that there was uncertainty about whether it would become a "classic pandemic."[32] You seem to make fun of "the readiness of so many to envisage the most far-reaching catastrophes."[33] That would be *me*, Susan. All bets were off. The CDC was lying about everything and not in a way that should have assured anyone that AIDS was not a "far-reaching catastrophe."

You wrote, "Everyone knows that a disproportionate number of blacks are getting AIDS,"[34] By who's definition of AIDS, Susan? The Vatican of public health? The CDC speaking ex cathedra?

You seemed to fancy yourself the linguistic AIDS police when you wrote, "This sort of rhetoric has a life of its own."[35] By making it seem like an apocalyptic vision of the epidemic is absurd and driven by some conservative political need for repression, you made it impossible to tell the truth about a pandemic without looking like a fascist hysteric, an enabler of right wing agendas.

How was one to do investigative reporting that undermined the CDC's credibility without being accused of what you called "end-of-the-world rhetoric"? You psychologize and gaslight those who did the critical thinking and the investigative reporting that uncovered a totally different epidemic from the one you were helping to sell to the public. From your literary throne you turned them into wacky conspiracy theorists when you wrote, "In the countdown to a millennium, a rise in apocalyptic thinking may be inevitable."[36] You talk about "fantasies of doom," an "imaginative complicity with disaster," and "apocalyptic rhetoric."[37] You really were the Gaslighter-in-Chief of the AIDS epidemic.

I think it is safe to say that, to a certain extent, your *AIDS and Its Metaphors* is one of the great works of bullshit of the twentieth century. You blame AIDS on the "mobility and interconnectedness (with its consequent dissolving of old taboos, social and sexual) [that] is as vital to the maximum functioning of the advanced, or world capitalist economy as is the easy transmissibility of goods and images and financial instruments."[38] OMG, Susan. Are you the Karl Marx of AIDS? And let me guess what *dissolved taboo* you were most concerned with.

You wanted to strip AIDS of all its apocalyptic metaphors and make it just a disease, just like any other. As though the problem of the epidemic lay in its discourse. Just think about it and talk about it differently and everything will be better. How about just telling the truth about it, no matter how horrifying, which is exactly what the CDC did *not* do! Scientific truth is not a metaphor problem, Susan. The power politics of science and public health are not a metaphor problem. They are a truthfulness-in-science-problem, a reality problem. A powerlessness-of-minorities problem.

You talk about the struggle for the "rhetorical ownership of the illness."[39] Well, I'll tell you one person who should never had any rhetorical ownership of the disease: Susan Sontag.

The primary ownership of the disease was in the hands of the CDC's white heterosexuals who had political and scientific power, otherwise known as public health epidemiology. Not gays or blacks. The primary institution that owned that rhetoric was the Centers for Disease Control. Silence about that is what equals death.

I came down to SoHo to try and convince you that the CDC was as honest during AIDS as it was during the Tuskegee Syphilis Experiment.

You said you wanted to "detach" the disease from "guilt and shame" and insisted that 'its disfiguring metaphors needed be exposed, criticized, belabored, used up."

But Susan, who gives a flying fuck about the disfiguring metaphor, the rhetoric, and language games if the discussion is grounded in the corrupt realpolitik of scientific and medical fraud? Susan, *AIDS and Its Metaphors* was just a case of garbage in, garbage out. CDC garbage in, Susan Sontag garbage out.

No thanks to you, *New York Native* stayed in business for another seven years after your book came out.

The picture I tried to paint for you about what was really going on at the CDC just got filled in more and more by *New York Native* in the years that followed. You were still in and out of New York, so your lack of awareness about what we were reporting must have been a very deliberate decision. *New York Native* was always on your local newsstand waiting for you to take a peek. At your own risk.

For the rest of the *New York Native*'s publishing life, our reporter, Neenyah Ostrom covered the evolving story of HHV-6 and its relationship to both AIDS and Chronic Fatigue Syndrome. Every new bit of research on Chronic Fatigue Syndrome which she covered suggested that it had a great deal in common with AIDS. They were Tweedledum and Tweedledee. One of the first Chronic Fatigue Syndrome researchers, a scientist named Paul Cheney, called Chronic Fatigue Syndrome AIDS-minor. When I heard that I suggested it was like pregnancy-minor. Some called it the mirror image of AIDS. One activist called it "Non-HIV AIDS."

I published three books by Neenyah Ostrom on the subject of Chronic Fatigue Syndrome and its relationship to the AIDS epidemic. One was called *What Really Killed Gilda Radner?* Gilda Radner had suffered from Chronic Fatigue Syndrome and had subsequently gotten a fatal case of cancer. Cancer was not an uncommon outcome of people who got Chronic Fatigue Syndrome. That was not surprising given the oncogenic nature of HHV-6, the dynamic and deadly virus that linked Chronic Fatigue Syndrome and AIDS.

The list of similarities between Chronic Fatigue Syndrome and AIDS is long and gets longer every day. All systems in the body are affected in Chronic Fatigue Syndrome. What happens in the brain is similar to AIDS. A whole list of secondary infections occurs, just like in AIDS. Even the dreaded Kaposi's Sarcoma virus has been found in Chronic Fatigue Syndrome patients.

The CDC didn't dare acknowledge these similarities. Worse, they would not even admit that Chronic Fatigue Syndrome is a real biological illness that is contagious and should be a notifiable infectious disease. While they turned a blind eye toward Chronic Fatigue Syndrome, it was allowed to spread and affect the lives of millions of people. Because of that, you could say that the real AIDS epidemic has not yet even begun. HIV-negative gay men have been dying at in an increased rate of illnesses that the CDC won't admit might be connected to the real epidemic of the HHV-6 family of viruses.

To add insult to injury, the CDC played around with the idea that Chronic Fatigue Syndrome was caused by traumatic events in childhood and was essentially a psychological disease that could be treated with some form of psychotherapeutic intervention. They would not accept the evidence that was emerging from published research or the words of the suffering patients. They essentially gaslighted both the evidence and the patients.

A pivotal moment in the cover-up of the relationship between Chronic Fatigue Syndrome and AIDS occurred at the International AIDS Conference that was held in Amsterdam in 1992. At that conference it was announced that AIDS-like illnesses were being seen in people who were *not infected with HIV*. It was the Black Swan moment when it should have been clear that HIV could not be the real cause of AIDS. The fact that some of the cases had also been diagnosed as Chronic Fatigue Syndrome cases should have made it clear that Chronic Fatigue Syndrome cases were part of the same epidemic and another agent they had in common should be considered as the possible cause of both supposedly different epidemics. And the leading suspect should have been the HHV-6 family of viruses.

But the CDC and the so-called AIDS Czar, Anthony Fauci, went into overdrive in their attempts to spin the dramatic findings in such a way that no such game-changing conclusions would be reached. In a classic case of circular reasoning, the CDC insisted that the cases were outliers, meaningless anomalies, and the fact that those affected with the AIDS-like illnesses weren't part of any risk group, proved that this was not really AIDS. Really? You could say that the closet door on the relationship between AIDS and Chronic Fatigue Syndrome was closed in Amsterdam. And nailed shut. Amsterdam was where Anthony Fauci's AIDS paradigm turned into a Bernie Madoff Ponzi scheme.

The hostility to my newspaper among true believers grew more and more intense as we raised doubts about the credibility of the CDC and the legitimacy of the HIV paradigm. The CDC and the NIH were annoyed with our coverage of the doubts about HIV and our reporting that exposed the links between Chronic Fatigue Syndrome, HHV-6, and AIDS. AIDS Czar Anthony Fauci even refused to shake the hand of one of my reporters at a news conference. The gay community began to turn on *New York Native*. Susan, even that friend who invited me to dinner with you took to viciously attacking me publicly. The media left us out on a limb. *The Village Voice*, that paragon of progressive thinking, published articles attacking *New York Native*. They published one article in which Larry Kramer said I should just shut up. That from a man whose historic essay I published and someone who inspired an organization whose mantra was "Silence equals death."

And then the AIDS activists started formally attacking *New York Native*. Most people think AIDS activists were fighting the government. But the truth is, they were totally behind the government's scientific dogma. The CDC, NIH, and Anthony Fauci made the AIDS activists their own Useful AIDS Idiots. They organized a boycott of *New York Native* that we somehow survived for a couple of years until we finally went under. We regularly delivered free copies of our newspaper to gay bars. During the boycott piles of them often ended up mysteriously in the trash. Try publishing a newspaper under those circumstances.

Susan, you defended Salman Rushdie when there was a Fatwa directed at him. But we couldn't depend on someone like you to defend our right to do investigative reporting on the cover-up of the relationship between Chronic Fatigue Syndrome and AIDS. You really were just an honorary member of

AIDS activist gang, haplessly, naively, doing the government's business.

When we went out of business in 1997, the media danced on our grave. Celebratory articles appeared in *New York Magazine*, *The New York Times* and the gay magazine called *The Advocate*. They made fun of our coverage of Chronic Fatigue Syndrome, HHV-6, and African Swine Fever.

In the years that followed, you wrote two successful novels which I took no interest in because you were no longer the Susan Sontag I thought you were. What did I feel when I heard you died of cancer in 2004? I don't know. Not what I felt when Hannah Arendt or Donna Summer died. Certainly not the sadness I would have felt if you had turned out to really be the inspiring, brilliant, and good person I thought you were when I fantasized about you in Kansas or interviewed you in New York in 1973, or spent that special night in Hell's Kitchen.

When I learned that you had died of a form of leukemia, I immediately did some research because I had a hunch, and that hunch turned out to be correct. Your cancer, Acute Myeloid Leukemia, which you fought so valiantly or insanely to the very end, was linked to HHV-6, the virus I had come to warn you about. You and Gilda Radner and millions of other people with cancer potentially related to the HHV-6 epidemic may have been in the same boat.

How is that for an apocalypse? Did anyone say "irony?" Believe me, you and Gilda Radner were just the tip of the HHV-6 cancer iceberg. Thanks to the CDC's cover-up of Chronic Fatigue Syndrome, millions of people are at risk for HHV-6 related cancers and other medical disasters.

Yes Susan, imagine that. Crazy isn't it? And you threw that newspaper that nailed the HHV-6 story and its publisher under the bus. Earth to Susan Sontag: You may have been a victim of the real epidemic. Yeah, that epidemic that mainly affected the poor folks with the vehement sexual customs and the voracious sexual appetites. The purveyors of "camp."

After you died, I was only left with the nagging mystery of why you had treated me the way you did in *AIDS and Its Metaphors*. Why had you screwed me? That question haunted me.

Until 2019.

That was the year that Benjamin Moser's seven-hundred-page biography of you came out. I got it from Amazon and read it immediately, stopping for breaks only to call friends about it. "You gotta buy this book. It's a total mindfuck," I told them all.

Mindfuck is an understatement.

Mr. Moser spent seven years reading almost every word you ever wrote—including your journals and your emails—and interviewed almost everyone you ever knew. He even had access to everything on your computer.

I say almost everyone, because, for some reason, he never tracked *me* down, and he never knew about the interview I did with you in the gay magazine *Out*. And he was unaware of the meeting I had with you in which I tried to prevent you from becoming a Useful AIDS Idiot.

Oh Susan, Susan, Susan! What a mess you were. What a twisted, sick little puppy. The Emperor truly had no clothes.

When I try to tell people about the train wreck of a woman portrayed in this brilliant biography, I don't know where to begin.

I can't believe you didn't destroy your all-too-revealing journals. What Mr. Moser found in them was a candy store of self-doubt, self-hate, and enough lesbian shame to destroy a thousand Gay Pride parades.

I had no idea about that because I was one of the blind New Yorkers who thought you had some kind of bisexy ambiguousness going on. At the very least, I thought that even if you were not exactly gay, you were gay-friendly. Susan, after reading Mr. Moser's biography of you, I think Vladimir Putin is gay-friendlier.

It wasn't just lesbian shame. As detailed in Mr. Moser's biography, your condescension and contempt for gay men was chilling. Years ago, a gay editor I knew shocked me when said he always thought you worked for the C.I.A. As off-the-wall as that sounded to me then, I can now comprehend why he thought you were never what you seemed to be, that there was always something else going on with you.

The Moser book helped me understand why you threw me and my gay newspaper under the bus. How could I ever hope that you would take me or *New York Native* seriously?

The Moser book made me rethink every moment I ever spent with you.

Now I no longer ponder why you accepted the CDC's sneering homophobic paradigm of AIDS which covered up the real epidemic of HHV-6 and Chronic Fatigue Syndrome.

What is so amazing about you is that from the journals which Mr. Moser quotes, you actually knew that you were fucked up.[40] Big time.

And reality *was* a serious problem for you. No wonder you said to me, "You've always been very real to me." I didn't know you had a basic problem with reality.

Mr. Moser notes in his book that in your journals, "a fear emerges that" you were "a liar, a fake, a fraud." Bingo. You seem to have had a gaslighting relationship with yourself.

Mr. Moser writes that you were afraid of "people who might see through her and discover her unworthiness, her ugliness, her lies." Well, welcome to your nightmare, Susan.

No matter how real I seemed to you that day in SoHo, it didn't keep you from mocking the reality-based journalism of my gay newspaper. Believe it or not, Susan, I was in the reality business.

How could you possibly take a gay newspaper seriously, you who referred to yourself in your journals as a "queer,"[41] a sickening term that has now been adopted by self-destructive fools in our community. I hope that is not another one of your legacies.

Mr. Moser seems as troubled by what he found in you as anyone who was mistreated by you. And there was, apparently a long line of people who you screwed cavalierly. I wasn't special, after all. It turns out I got the classic Susan Sontag treatment.

The two big reveals in Mr. Moser's book, which seemed to help him understand what made you tick, are the fact that you were the classic dysfunctional adult child of an alcoholic[42] and if that isn't enough, you took amphetamines for twenty-five years.[43] You were a speed freak.

Who knew?

The hot mess of your nature turned Moser from biographer into diagnostician. But I think his diagnosis might not be on the money

I think there was something else going on. Something more basic and neurological. Mr. Moser gave us seven hundred pages of biographical dots that I would connect differently. As I read Mr. Moser's troubling account of you, the book that kept coming to mind was *Confessions of a Sociopath* by M.E. Thomas. I actually think you may have been wired like a sociopath. A highly-functioning, very self-aware, very literary sociopath. Not a criminal sociopath—except for some minor shoplifting, an incident of academic fraud, and a bit of alleged plagiarism. But someone who hurt a lot of people thoughtlessly and did a lot of damage. I mean *really* thoughtlessly. Something was obviously very developed in your brain. But something else was very *undeveloped*, or nonexistent in your brain. You were not wired for love or empathy. You were not wired to easily see what was going on around you.

You were what could be called a meta-sociopath, someone who explored their own fuckedupness regularly in their journals. Your fraudulent and complicated self fascinated you. I think you were a toxic stew of intelligence, ambition, pretentiousness, heartlessness, self-disgust, and raging narcissism. That's the *queer* reality that lurked beneath your legendary beauty and genius. I will hand you this. Your life was not boring and it made for one of the most interesting biographies I've ever read. But your life also offers a dramatic cautionary tale about the toxicity of homophobia and auto-homophobia.

The sociopathic tip-offs in your history and journals are pretty obvious. You knew you had a problem with empathy. You were convinced you could *become* empathetic,[44] but Susan, really? Sociopaths can't become what are called empaths just by an act of will. They certainly can *act* like they are empathetic. The best of them can put on the mask of empathy. Suddenly, your obsession with masks in the interview I did with you in 1973 made sense.

The way you used people, threw them overboard, humiliated so-called lovers and friends throughout Mr. Moser's cinematic biography can't help but make one think of sociopathology. Something hardwired was going on. There was malware in your soul. Even your failure to bathe or brush your teeth, and your odd reputation for eating grotesquely as recounted in the Moser biography, says there was something neurological going on with you. Words like "weirdo," or "eccentric" just won't cut it.

Of all the upsetting stories in the book, the one I will never get out of my head is the one in which you would often call your celebrated partner Annie Lebovitz stupid in front of people at dinner parties in Manhattan. Annie Lebovitz, stupid? WTF? I guess you didn't get very far in empathy 101.

It turns out that AIDS was not the only issue you had terrible judgment about. Mr. Moser reminds us that your young, glib, Marxist self could muster only minor concern about the way gay people were being treated—I should say tortured—in Cuba, when you wrote your laudatory piece about the Cuban revolution.[45] And the piece you wrote from Hanoi praising the government of North Vietnam was oblivious to the fact that a couple of blocks away from where you were, American soldiers were being tortured in a hotel.[46] And your piece on China seemed to lack any serious empathy for those who suffered the consequences of totalitarianism.[47]

Yes, there were a handful of things you did well in your life, even nobly—at least on the public relations surface. But one troubling question will always stalk your history. What was real and what was an act? When were you not a fraud?

According to Mr. Moser, near the end of your life you gave an interview to Joan Acocella of *The New Yorker* in which she pressed you on your personal life. Even though everyone on the New York City grapevine knew about your relationship with Annie Lebovitz, you had to be dragged kicking and screaming into admitting you had relationships with *men and women.*[48]

Mr. Moser noted that in your journals you wrote that you experienced "the incipient guilt I have always felt about my lesbianism—making me ugly to myself" and "Being queer makes me feel more vulnerable. It increases my wish to hide, to be invisible."[49]

Mr. Moser points out that in your novel, *The Benefactor,* being homosexual is synonymous with being phony" and "Gay people are not real people but caricatures playing roles" and "Homosexuality is phoniness, theater, a means of attracting attention."[50]

When you decided in your youth to become heterosexual, or heterosexualish, it seemed like you devised your own personal gay conversion therapy program, forcing yourself to sleep with men and ultimately get married.

According to Moser, your ex-husband thought homosexuals were "disgusting. Love for them was impossible."[51] Was your husband's take on it that different from what *you* thought? I don't think the apple fell far from the marriage.

Susan, according to Mr. Moser, you were mesmerized early in your life by the Djuna Barnes novel, *Nightwood*. He quotes a passage from it about lesbianism that foreshadows your own take on the subject: "Like the poor beasts that get their antlers mixed and are found dead that way, their heads fattened with a knowledge of each other that they never wanted, having had to contemplate, head-on and eye-to-eye, until death."[52] Now whenever I think of you Susan, I will think of antlers and dead lesbians.

Your assistant, Karla Eoff, told Mr. Moser that when she urged you to admit you were bisexual, you said to her, "I don't think same-sex relationships are valid," and "The parts don't fit."[53]

Moser notes that you felt like you were slumming your whole life.[54] Were you slumming when I interviewed you, when I spent what I thought was a magical night with you, and most importantly, when I came down to SoHo as a besieged journalist begging for help?

As I have written in all of my books, homophobia lies at the core of the cover-up of the truth about AIDS, HHV-6 and the Chronic Fatigue Syndrome epidemic. I have also described the pseudo-science of the epidemic as "sociopathic science," science that demeans and deceives the very people it is supposed to be helping. Science that covertly victimizes and does not have empathy for its victims.

(*Susan gets up and moves toward the front of the stage toward OLD ORTLEB. They stand two feet apart staring at each other*)

So, Susan, in some ways you were the perfect person to write about the epidemic. You made an excellent Useful AIDS Idiot. Homophobia and auto-homophobia are fertile ground for the development of Useful AIDS Idiots. You once wrote, "The writer's first job is not to have opinions but to tell the truth . . . and refuse to be an accomplice of lies and misinformation."[55] That beautifully describes what you were *not* doing when you wrote about AIDS. Nor does it describe all the poems, movies, and plays that were written by the CDC's other celebrated Useful AIDS Idiots. Even the ones that succeeded on Broadway with normal hearts, angels, E.M. Forster, or whatever.

The sociopathic Useful AIDS Idiot paradigm you enabled and helped polish exists to this very day. The apocalyptic HHV-6 epidemic remains hidden in plain sight. The CDC continues to pretend that Chronic Fatigue Syndrome isn't an epidemic and isn't the other face of the AIDS epidemic. And the family of HHV-6 viruses is treated like it is ubiquitous but harmless. You and all of the Useful AIDS Idiots have been very useful. The CDC and the NIH salute you.

But what do I know Susan? Your former adoring acolyte was just the gay publisher of a gay newspaper. I was part of a minority that isn't valid. I was a caricature playing a role.

The world will have to decide. History will have to choose sides. Let everyone read our books. Let them study what is in *New York Native*. One of us is full of shit. Is it me? Is it you? Let society and history judge. The future of public health may depend upon which one of us is right. (*Walks up to her.*) Am I still very real to you? (*He hands her the white rose.*)

SUSAN SONTAG. (*She takes the rose, looks at it and then at him.*) You don't miss a thing, do you?

Curtain

Afterword

In the mid-1990s, as publisher of *New York Native*, I urged Congressman Jerold Nadler and his staff to look into the CDC's mishandling of Chronic Fatigue Syndrome and the possible cover-up of its relationship to the AIDS epidemic and HHV-6. As a result, he sent this letter to the Secretary of Health and Human Services.

April 12, 1996

The Honorable Donna E. Shalala
Secretary of Health and Human Services
200 Independence Avenue SW
Washington, D.C. 20202

Dear Secretary Shalala,

A very serious charge has been made by author Hillary Johnson that the Centers for Disease Control (CDC) have covered up the existence of a significant public health issue Chronic Fatigue Syndrome (CFS). Ms. Johnson has asserted in her recent book, *Osler's Web*, as well as in interviews and public appearances on *Good Morning America* and other major venues that CFS is a real disease caused by a real pathogen, but that the CDC has attempted to portray CFS as a psychosomatic illness instead. She alleges that CFS is a major debilitating illness with enormous public health consequences. In over 720 pages, based on 9 years of investigation, she sets out to prove that CFS is an infectious disease that attacks the brain and leaves its victims totally devastated.

Ms. Johnson asserts that there is already ample clinical and epidemiological evidence to support her conclusion, but CDC is hidebound in its determination to ignore this evidence—at the public's peril. She believes the CDC refuses to draw the obvious conclusion from the evidence because of a handful of longtime CDC senior scientists and other scientists have attempted to draw the same conclusions that she has have been ostracized and denied federal funding.

This matter was initially brought to my attention because of Ms. Johnson assertion that CFS is an immunological disease with many of the same characteristics as AIDS. In fact, on page 33 of her book, she calls CFS "HIV-negative AIDS." In Chapter 27 (492-493), Ms. Johnson briefly discusses research regarding the possibility that the herpesvirus HHV-6 may be the causative agent or a contributing player in the development and symptoms of CFS. In Chapter 33, she reports that HHV-6 may be involved as a precipitating factor in other immunological illnesses, including AIDS.

Because of the implications for public health if Ms. Johnson assertions turn out to be true and because of their serious impact on the public's confidence in the CDC, Ms. Johnson's allegations about CFS deserve the most immediate and serious attention. I ask that you personally look into this matter.

Sincerely,

JERROLD NADLER

Member of Congress

Congressman Nadler read this statement on the Floor of Congress on April 16, 1996.

I have learned of a serious charge made by author Hillary Johnson in her book Osler's Web, that the CDC has ignored clinical and epidemiological evidence that Chronic Fatigue Syndrome (CFS) is a devastating infectious disease caused by a real pathogen, rather than a psychosomatic illness as the CDC has claimed. Ms. Johnson charges that researchers who share her view have been ostracized and denied federal funding.

She asserts that CFS is an immunological disease with many of the same characteristics as AIDS. She calls CFS "HIV-Negative AIDS" and reports the view of some others that HHV-6 may be a precipitating factor or a co-factor in CFS and other immunological illnesses, including AIDS.

I have already contacted HHS Secretary Shalala requesting her response to Ms. Johnson's disturbing allegations and I now urge that Congress direct the GAO to look into this matter as well.

In the December, 2009, issue of *Journal of Virology*, a group of scientists at Washington University School of Medicine published a paper titled "Detection of novel sequences related to African Swine Fever virus in human serum and sewage." The scientists concluded that "Detection of these sequences [related to African Swine Fever virus] suggests that greater genetic diversity may exist among asfarviruses than previously thought and raises the possibility that human infection by asfarviruses may occur." They also asserted, "Although ASFV is not known to infect humans even where the virus is endemic, identification of ASFV-like sequences in serum from multiple human patients suggests that human infection may occur."

On May 24, 2017, HHV-6 University published "The HHV-6 Declaration of the Rights of Man."

1. The right not to be lied to about the role of HHV-6 in AIDS.

2. The right not to be lied to about the role of HHV-6 in Chronic Fatigue Syndrome.

3. The right not to be lied to about the role of HHV-6 in Autism.

4. The right not to be lied to about the role of HHV-6 in Multiple Sclerosis.

5. The right not to be lied to about the role of HHV-6 in Brain Cancer.

6. The right not to be lied to about the role of HHV-6 in Heart Disease.

7. The right not to be lied to about the role of HHV-6 in Encephalitis.

8. The right not to be lied to about the role of HHV-6 in Cognitive Dysfunction.

9. The right not to be lied to about the role of HHV-6 in Drug Hypersensitivity Syndrome.

10. The right not to be lied to about the role of HHV-6 in Bone Marrow Suppression.

11. The right not to be lied to about the role of HHV-6 in Lymphadenopathy.

12. The right not to be lied to about the role of HHV-6 in Colitis.

13. The right not to be lied to about the role of HHV-6 in Endocrine Disorders.

14. The right not to be lied to about the role of HHV-6 in Liver Disease.

15. The right not to be lied to about the role of HHV-6 in Hodgkin's Lymphoma.

16. The right not to be lied to about the role of HHV-6 in Glioma.

17. The right not to be lied to about the role of HHV-6 in Cervical Cancer.

18. The right not to be lied to about the role of HHV-6 in Hypogammaglobulinemia.

19. The right not to be lied to about the role of HHV-6 in Optic Neuritis.

20. The right not to be lied to about the role of HHV-6 in Microangiopathy.

21. The right not to be lied to about the role of HHV-6 in Mononucleosis.

22. The right not to be lied to about the role of HHV-6 in Uveitis.

23. The right not to be lied to about the role of HHV-6 in Stevens-Johnson Syndrome.

24. The right not to be lied to about the role of HHV-6 in Rhomboencephalitis.

25. The right not to be lied to about the role of HHV-6 in Limbic Encephalitis.

26. The right not to be lied to about the role of HHV-6 in Encephalomyelitis

27. The right not to be lied to about the role of HHV-6 in Pneumonitis.

28. The right not to be lied to about the role of HHV-6 in GVHD.

29. The right not to be lied to about the role of HHV-6 in Ideopathic Pneumonia.

30. The right not to be lied to about the role of HHV-6 in Pediatric Adrenocortical Tumors

31. The right not to be lied to about the role of HHV-6 in the reactivation of endogenous retroviruses.

32. The right not to be lied to about the impact of HHV-6 on T-Cells.

33. The right not to be lied to about the impact of HHV-6 on B-Cells

34. The right not to be lied to about the impact of HHV-6 on Epithelial Cells.

35. The right not to be lied to about the impact of HHV-6 on Natural Killer Cells.

36. The right not to be lied to about the impact of HHV-6 on Dendritic Cells.

37. The right not to be lied to about the impact of HHV-6 infection of the brain.

38. The right not to be lied to about the impact of HHV-6 infection of the liver.

39. The right not to lied to about the ability of HHV-6 to affect cytokine production.

40. The right not to be lied to about the ability of HHV-6 to affect Aortic and Heart Microvascular Endothelial cells.

41. The right not to be lied to about the role of an HHV-6 cover-up in a massive HIV Fraud Ponzi Scheme that in a number of ways resembles the Tuskegee Syphilis Experiment and Nazi medicine.

On September 14, 2018 The University of Wurzburg issued this statement: "While HHV-6 was long believed to have no negative impact on human health, scientists today increasingly suspect the virus of causing various diseases such as multiple sclerosis or chronic fatigue syndrome. Recent studies even suggest that HHV-6 might play a role in the pathogenesis of several diseases of the central nervous system such as schizophrenia, bipolar disorder, depression or Alzheimer's."

https://www.uni-wuerzburg.de/en/news-and-events/news/detail/news/viruses-under-the-microscope/

On November 20, 2018, HHV-6 University named Bhupesh Prusty Scientist of the Year for his research showing that HHV-6 is playing a major role in Chronic Fatigue Syndrome.

On January 27, 2019, on the HHV-6 University website, I called for the creation of a CFS/AIDS New Deal:

The CFS/AIDS New Deal calls for equal funding for Chronic Fatigue Syndrome and AIDS research, treatment, and prevention, and that they be researched side-by-side to determine if they are one epidemic.

On November 14, 2019, African Swine Fever University reported that Cooper Farms veterinarian Don Davidson had told *Food Safety News* that he thought that African Swine Fever was probably already in North America.

On November 27, 2019, HHV-6 University named Anna Fogdell-Hahne the scientist of the year for her work linking HHV-6 to Multiple Sclerosis.

Books by Charles Ortleb Available on Amazon.

Apocalypse Then and Now: Collected Works 1980-2020

The Chronic Fatigue Syndrome Epidemic Cover-up: How a Little Newspaper Solved the Biggest Scientific and Political Mystery of Our Time

The Chronic Fatigue Syndrome Epidemic Cover-up Volume Two: The Origins of Totalitarianism in Science and Medicine

Fauci: The Bernie Madoff of Science and the HIV Ponzi Scheme that Concealed the Chronic Fatigue Syndrome Epidemic

Iatrogenocide: Notes for a Political Philosophy of Epidemiology and Science.

Patient Zero: Why the 1980 cases of Chronic Fatigue Syndrome in Atlanta should have been recognized as the other face of the AIDS epidemic.

The Closing Argument: A shocking courtroom novella about AIDS, Chronic Fatigue Syndrome, racial injustice and HHV-6, the virus that threatens us all

The Stonewall Massacre

The African Swine Fever Novel

The Black Party: A Dramatic Comedy in Two Acts

The Last Lovers on Earth: Stories from Dark Times

Iron Peter: A Year in the Mythopoetic Life of New York City

Butterfly Ghosts and The New Hippocratic Oath: Earlier and Later Poems

Charles Ortleb Presents the P-hacking Cartoons of Julian Lake: A Humorous Look at the Fraudulent and Unethical Culture of Chronic Fatigue Syndrome and AIDS Research

Notes

[1] Susan Sontag, *Illness as Metaphor and AIDS and Its Metaphors*, (New York : Picador, 2002) p.102.

[2] Ibid., p. 109.

[3] Ibid, p.112.

[4] Ibid., p. 113.

[5] Ibid.

[6] Ibid.

[7] Ibid., p. 114.

[8] Ibid.

[9] Ibid.

[10] Ibid., p. 115.

[11] Ibid., p.116.

[12] Ibid., p. 119.

[13] Ibid., p. 121.

[14] Ibid.

[15] Ibid., p. 125.

[16] Ibid., p. 134.

[17] Ibid., p. 140.

[18] Ibid., p. 141.

[19] Ibid, p. 142.

[20] Ibid., p. 144.

[21] Ibid.

[22] Ibid., p. 146.

[23] Ibid., p. 146.

[24] Ibid., p. 158.

[25] Ibid., p. 160.

[26] Ibid.

[27] Ibid., p. 161.

[28] Ibid., p. 164.

[29] Ibid., p. 165

[30] Ibid., p. 166.

[31] Ibid., 168.

[32] Ibid., p. 170

[33] Ibid.
[34] Ibid.
[35] Ibid., p. 173.
[36] Ivid., p. 175.
[37] Ibid., p. 175.
[38] Ibid., p. 180.
[39] Iid., p. 181.
[40] Benjamin Moser, Sontag: Her Life and Her Work (New York: Harper Collins, 2019) p. 70.
[41] Ibid., p. 76
[42] Ibid., p. 194
[43] Ibid, p. 455
[44] Ibid., p. 164
[45] Ibid., p. 326.
[46] Ibid., p. 305
[47] Ibid., p. 340.
[48] Ibid., p. 631
[49] Ibid., p. 75.
[50] Ibid., p. 196
[51] Ibid., p. 129.
[52] Ibid., p. 84.
[53] Ibid., p. 628.
[54] Ibid., p. 59.
[55] *Susan Sontag (2007). "At the Same Time: Essays and Speeches", p.193, Macmillan*

www.ingramcontent.com/pod-product-compliance
Lightning Source LLC
Chambersburg PA
CBHW030948240526
45463CB00016B/2070